Naked
at Our
Age

Naked at Our Age

Talking Out Loud About Senior Sex

JOAN PRICE

Foreword by Betty Dodson

SEAL PRESS

Naked at Our Age
Talking Out Loud About Senior Sex

Copyright © 2011 by Joan Price

Published by
Seal Press
A Member of the Perseus Books Group
1700 Fourth Street
Berkeley, California

Library of Congress Cataloging-in-Publication Data

Price, Joan, 1943-
  Naked at our age : talking out loud about senior sex / Joan Price.
    p. cm.
  Includes index.
  ISBN 978-1-58005-338-9
  1. Older people--Sexual behavior. I. Title.
  HQ30.P75 2011
  613.9'5--dc22

                                        2010033379

10 9 8 7

Cover design by Domini Dragoone
Interior design by Megan Jones Design
Printed in the United States of America
Distributed by Publishers Group West

Naked at Our Age *is dedicated to the memory of my beloved husband, Robert Rice. Although Robert died before this book could be written, it is as much his as mine. "You honor me when you do your work," I hear his voice tell me. So, Robert, this book is for you, in your honor, with memories of our great love.*

CONTENTS

FOREWORD
by Betty Dodson, PhD

JOAN PRICE HAS written an informative book about a much maligned group, sexual seniors. Many believe that sex for old people is nonexistent, disgusting, or downright laughable. But all you folks can wipe those grins of embarrassment off your face and accept this as a fact: American seniors are living well into their eighties today and many of us are still self-sufficient and very much interested in sustaining sexual activity. It's time for everyone to accept that, if they're lucky, they too will be old someday. And if they make it, most will want to have some form of sexual expression.

Throughout my life, most of my thoughts, conversations, drawings, articles, and books have centered on sexual themes. In spite of the advantages that come with years of focusing on the erotic realm, remaining a sexually active senior has required a concerted effort. Aging with style has taken a lot of courage, along with a robust sense of humor. I no longer care what people will think, and I don't worry about making a fool of myself. Instead, I continue to live my life out loud and sex-proud at every age.

Masturbation is the foundation for all of human sexuality. It is our first natural sexual activity; it's the way we learn to like our genitals and it's how we discover sexual pleasure. Once masturbation enters the lexicon of human sexuality and is properly honored, we will move into a new phase of social harmony within ourselves, our relationships, our families, and the global community.

As OUR BODIES change, so does our ability to have sex with a partner. You'll find a detailed discussion about this in Joan's book. Even sex with ourselves changes, but it rarely goes away if a person has enjoyed a relatively active sex life of some kind. For those of us who have spent a large part of our adult lives enjoying different aspects of sex, we will manage to find ways to continue to do so.

In the early 1980s, when I turned fifty, I went into menopause. Margaret Mead described older women as having a "postmenopausal zest" with a renewed energy and strength to devote to a commitment in their chosen field or creative project. Instead of fearing this change and seeing it as the end of my fertile years, which meant I'd be less desirable in the sexual realm, I saw menopause as a new beginning.

As I approached sixty, I felt a need to challenge the aging process more assertively. My hip joints were getting stiff and painful, and I was faced with a physical challenge. Some days I was nearly crippled. When my hip pain had progressed to the place that I couldn't comfortably open my legs to make room for a partner to penetrate me, I opted for bilateral hip replacement surgery at the age of sixty-seven. A year later I was a born-again hedonist.

One of the most important things I learned about senior partner sex is taking turns. This allows each person to fully focus on building up sexual arousal to orgasm. For me to have an orgasm, I must put my total attention on my own body and sensations. This is seldom discussed because we continue to act as though partner sex is something that comes naturally instead of being a complicated art form that requires skill and practice. Today, partner-assisted masturbation is one of my favorite forms of sharing orgasms. Or I'll use a vibrator on my clitoris during intercourse. Vaginal penetration is often his end pleasure, but for me it's just a beginning.

FOR THE RECORD, most young and older men have no complaints when a woman states her sexual preferences. If anything, they are relieved when she is clear about what she wants. After all, sex is adult play, and it's no fun if we inhibit our pleasure by pretending what works for a partner works for us too.

The decade of my seventies, which I see as the youth of old age, was far more delightful than I could have imagined. It was some of my best partner sex ever—with a man who was in his twenties! I wrote about this ten-year affair in *Orgasms for Two: The Joy of Partnersex*.

Now, as a single woman again at the age of eighty-one, I'm very aware of my aging body with brown spots cropping up all over, my round belly pulling on my lower back creating pain, and all that wrinkled skin. That's when I remember to count my blessings. I can still walk, talk, laugh, sing, dance, write, and have an orgasm any time I desire with one of my many vibrators and a fantasy. I love my website with Carlin Ross, www.dodsonand ross.com, where I answer sex questions for people from around the world. My background as an artist and PhD sexologist dovetails nicely with Carlin, who was formerly a lawyer and a brilliant cyber geek.

While we can all agree with Bette Davis, who said, "Old Age ain't for sissies," no one tells us the good news about growing older, like the freedom that comes with knowledge, no longer caring what people think, and enjoying the fruits of our labors.

I see aging as the final challenge. Instead of a Grim Reaper who waits in the shadows to whisk us off to some dark scary unknown place, I prefer to see death as my final work of art, the ultimate orgasm being when the life force leaves my body. Until then, I'll continue to figure out ways to enjoy my older body. As long as I can access my mind for sexual memories and fantasies while I hold a vibrator on my clitoris for one more orgasm, I'm here for the long haul as I head for one hundred or more.

Let Joan's book inspire you to enjoy your sex life to the end.

BETTY DODSON, PH.D.
NEW YORK CITY, 2010
WWW.DODSONANDROSS.COM

INTRODUCTION

I STARTED WRITING ABOUT senior sex after falling in love, at age fifty-seven, with the love of my life, artist Robert Rice (yes, his last name differed from mine by one letter), who was then sixty-four. We gloried in our close connection, our spicy and exhilarating sexuality.

Our sexy love story propelled me to write a candid book celebrating senior sex: *Better Than I Ever Expected: Straight Talk about Sex After Sixty,* published by Seal Press in 2006. I was on a mission: It was time for our generation to talk out loud about senior sexuality and prove that wrinkles and decades of birthdays are no deterrent to hot sex.

I spoke at bookstores, women-friendly sexuality shops, senior expos, even a naturist resort where many in my audience sat nude (I stayed dressed). As I traveled and met new people, two common themes kept coming up. Women and men started saying to me, "Well, bully for you for having such great sex, but I'm not, and here's why . . ." And men in the audience told me, "*Better Than I Ever Expected* is for women. What about us? Where's the book addressing our concerns?"

I realized that I had to write a new book about senior sex, this time addressing both women and men, and this time dealing with their problems head-on. I solicited interviews from boomers, seniors, and elders who had sexual concerns related to aging. I rewrote the questionnaire I had used for *Better Than I Ever Expected*, concentrating on the problems more than the delights. I emailed this questionnaire to readers who had contacted me already, and solicited more interviews on my blog, other blogs read by the age fifty-plus community, and at my talks and workshops. In the questionnaire, I asked interviewees to answer in detail any question that applied to them and ignore the rest, or to just tell their story in their own way. I promised confidentiality— they would choose a "code name" (a first name of their choice) and no one but me would know their true identities.

Questionnaires poured in from both women and men, sharing intimate details that sometimes even their partners didn't know. People really wanted to share their stories and ask questions. They needed help and information.

As I read the questionnaires, I started making a list of the topics that kept coming up and which interviews related to which topics. Then I pulled excerpts from each questionnaire and turned them into the reader's "story," keeping the interviewee's personal style and wording.

I didn't personally know the answer to every question, but I knew where to find it. I contacted experts in the field, asking them to respond to the issues that kept coming up. Some of these experts were specialized—dealing with sexuality and cancer, erectile dysfunction, or vaginal pain, for example. Others were counselors or sex therapists who dealt with a range of issues. I matched the experts with particular stories, and their responses became the information and advice in each chapter.

And a new book was born. Each chapter addresses a particular, age-related sexual concern, and includes both stories from the questionnaires and expert tips.

I WAS WORKING on this book when Robert—whose leukemia and lymphoma were in remission after chemotherapy—was diagnosed with a new cancer: multiple myeloma. This cancer affects the bone marrow's ability to produce healthy blood. I put the book on hold and concentrated on loving Robert, exploring medical options, keeping him close, and treasuring the moments we had left.

Robert experienced extreme fatigue. His fragile bones broke, and as treatments failed, he aged and weakened before my eyes. But almost to the end, he and I kept talking about this book: what would be in it, and why it was important to write it, no matter what happened in our personal lives. He said earnestly many times, "Promise me you'll keep doing your work."

Robert died in August 2008. I catapulted into extreme grief and depression. I kept collecting interviews but basically put the book on hold for more than a year. I couldn't concentrate enough to work, though my promise to Robert stayed in my mind.

Sometimes I heard Robert's voice guiding me, comforting me. One day he seemed to say gently, "I don't want to be the reason you're not living your life." I decided that I needed to get back to work on this book.

I am happy and proud to share it with you here.

Naked at Our Age: Talking Out Loud About Senior Sex is a candid, straight-talking book addressing senior sexuality in all its colors: the challenges, the disappointments, and the surprises, as well as the delights and the love stories. *Naked at Our Age* gives real-life people, age fifty to ninety, a voice to tell stories of their past and present sex lives, ask questions, and get straightforward advice and information. No topic related to elder sexuality is off-limits.

Women and men, coupled and single, straight and gay, talk candidly here about how their sex lives and relationships have changed with age, and about how they see themselves, their partners, or their single life. Many of the people featured in this book are having unsatisfying sex, or no sex, and are seeking solutions—help that sex therapists, health professionals, counselors, and other experts featured in this book have so generously provided. To learn more about the people giving advice in the book, turn to the Meet Our Experts section, in the back.

Naked at Our Age addresses the myriad changes in body and mind that affect sexuality. The stories people sent me reveal that what affects our sexuality isn't one single medical issue, hormonal concern, or marital conflict. Many physical and psychological dimensions create the ups and downs in our sexual response and satisfaction. The older we get, the more one change shapes another. A bad back, or prostate cancer, or a late-life divorce, for example, influences our mood, self-image, communication with a partner, and body experience, as well as sexual response. *Naked at Our Age* is not just a book on sexuality—it's a book about life force, about rebounding from life's challenges to keep on loving.

I love to hear from readers. I hope you'll email me (joan@joan price.com) and read my sex and aging blog, www.NakedAtOur Age.com, where we're keeping the conversation going.

JOAN PRICE
SEBASTOPOL, CALIFORNIA

1

The Old Ways Don't Do It Anymore!

W E SPEND OUR twenties and thirties grounding ourselves, sexually. Then that ground starts to shift in our forties and fifties, and, for many of us, a major landslide begins in our sixties and seventies. Our bodies, sexual responses, and relationships begin changing and don't always work the way they used to.

But with self-knowledge, creativity, good communication, and a sense of humor, we can roll with the changes and make the earth move again. Sex might not feel or look the way it did when our hormone rush propelled us into jet-stream sex, but it can be highly arousing and satisfying.

This chapter offers tips for general age-related sex and relationship problems. The chapters that follow address specific problems in detail.

Working with What Works . . . and Talking about It

A woman wrote me, "Having my breasts touched used to arouse me, but now I hate it." She described how her husband "mauled" her breasts, and how she turned off completely. Shortly after that, a man emailed me, writing, "My wife always liked having her breasts touched, but now, no matter how much I do it, she doesn't seem turned on."

I don't know for sure that these two were husband and wife, but it fits. She couldn't tell him that she didn't want her breasts touched now, and he thought he just wasn't doing it enough. The moral of the story: Talk to each other!

Many times, communication breaks down when the old ways don't work anymore. We don't want to hurt or offend a partner who's trying so hard to give us pleasure, so we might not start a conversation about what we need now. But we need to communicate to our partner how we're experiencing sensation differently. When we don't, our partner is likely to keep doing the same thing, not knowing it doesn't work anymore.

But sometimes we don't even *know* what works for us anymore, and we have to figure out all over again what arouses and satisfies us. Sensations change, and we may be more or less sensitive in the parts we always counted on to arouse us. We may need more foreplay. We may be more aroused by oral play than intercourse. We may need the addition of sex toys to reach orgasm. The best way to figure out what works is to experiment with pleasuring ourselves solo. (See Chapter 8.)

As long as we can communicate intimately and honestly with our partner about what turns us on and what turns us off, we can navigate the many changes and issues we may be dealing with. Here's how some of us have resolved this:

CLAIRE, AGE 56

At my age, my agility and stamina challenge me in a sexual situation. I inform my partner, "Gee, I just can't do that," and we laugh and try something else. It's okay, there are lots of ways to achieve the same pleasurable result. It's not necessary for me to raise my legs up over my ears! I love to be fingered by my lover. Many men regard digital manipulation as either unnecessary or just something they do quickly to get things moist enough to shove their dick in. So when I find a lover who will spend time pleasuring me with his fingers, I feel very lucky.

SANDY, AGE 51

My husband starts setting up between one and six hours before we will get intimate. He knows that I take a long time to get aroused, so he will rent a porn DVD or find a porn website for me to watch. When I watch porn on the computer, he gets under the table and performs oral sex on me. I have experienced up to three orgasms in a matter of minutes this way.

JAKE, AGE 54

I get turned on the most by arousing my wife and giving her sexual pleasure. I love it when I'm able to help her achieve a satisfying orgasm. She doesn't climax very easily, so when it does happen, it's a welcome event for both of us. Sometimes when she climaxes, her contractions continue on and on until she has to stop the stimulation because it's just too much for her. Once she recovers, she opens herself up for me and begs me to "bump" her, as she puts it. Of course I comply willingly and allow my body's instincts to take over, knowing that my own pent-up climax that I've been deliberately holding back is not far away.

ADVICE FROM AN EXPERT
Changing Tastes
BY CAROL QUEEN, PHD

Sexuality is fluid, and yours may be changing. What kind of sex you like best, how long it takes to get turned on, how long you like it to last, what you fantasize, the qualities of your preferred partner(s), including gender—*everything* that makes a difference to your erotic experience is individual and subject to change.

It might take longer to come to orgasm, the vagina may not lubricate as much, and certain positions can be unkind to your hips or knees. But other things may cause a shift in your own self-image or identity—like whether you desire women or men or both, or whether you want to initiate versus waiting to be approached by your partner, or if you decide it's time to try things you've never tried before. If the old, reliable sexual elements feel less interesting now, it may simply mean you have new interests ready to take their places—or would, if you open your mind to them.

Major sexual changes *can* be caused by the onset of serious illness and are a reason to get a checkup. Doctors can evaluate you for diabetes, depression, neurological problems, heart and other circulatory issues, and other conditions that might affect your sex drive and enjoyment. I encourage you to mention your sexual issues to your doctor, though many doctors will not have the knowledge and resources to deal specifically with sexual concerns. For sexual issues related to knowledge and behaviors, not physical health, a clinical sexologist or a sex therapist will be best able to help.

GORDON, AGE 58

My enjoyment of sex is variable and problematic these days. The big problem is physical unreliability. In my young days, sex was rarely anything but great in terms of my physical functioning. Nowadays, sex is occasionally as good as ever, but it is often rather lackluster. I rarely have trouble getting an erection, but sometimes it deflates a bit just before climax. Other times the orgasm is drab, even if I maintain my erection.

My partner has a lot of trouble achieving orgasm. I am not sure that I have ever given her one. She says that it requires breast and clitoral stimulation simultaneously. She clearly enjoys our sex without having orgasms, and since she says she is satisfied with it, I do not see any big problem. I mean that I don't feel any requirement to go all out to try to bring her to orgasm, but I would very much like to do it occasionally. Once in a long while I try, but she usually stops me after a short time. I would like to understand this part of her sexuality better.

I grew up with one belief that I know was naive—that sex should come naturally; that men in particular should not have to learn anything about sex. While being sexual does come naturally at a basic level, there is a huge amount of practical education that one can learn only in bed, and different women like very different things. I have been able to deeply satisfy a few women, but a few others have found me lacking. I think I could still learn a lot about sex.

An Expert Responds
MICHAEL CASTLEMAN, MA

Gordon, you say that your lover has difficulty experiencing orgasm, and that you don't feel it's your responsibility to "go all out to bring her to orgasm." You're right . . . to a point. No one "gives" anyone an orgasm. Orgasms are like laughter. They emerge from within us when conditions are right. Comedians can be funny, but they don't "make" us laugh. They simply provide the context for us to allow laughter to emerge from deep within us. Orgasms are similar. It's not your responsibility to bring her to orgasm. It is your responsibility to create the context that allows her to feel sufficiently relaxed, comfortable, and loved to let one out.

It's possible that she doesn't care if she comes or not. But if she wants orgasms, your stated indifference to her coming may be interfering with her ability to get there. Give her what she enjoys. She likes simultaneous breast and clitoral stimulation. It's no sacrifice on your part to fondle or suckle her nipple while gently caressing her clitoris, and to provide oral sex while your hands gently caress her breasts.

If extended breast-and-clitoral stimulation doesn't do it for her, incorporate a vibrator into your lovemaking. After you caress her breasts and clitoris for a long, relaxed time, hold her in a loving embrace while she uses a vibrator to have an orgasm. You might study how she uses the vibe, and then, with her coaching, use it on her yourself.

You mention that your own pleasure is flagging; that it's less reliable. For "drab" orgasms, I suggest you try Kegel exercises, which tone the pelvic floor muscles that contract during orgasm. I bet that if you practice Kegels a few times a day for three months, you'll notice more pleasure in orgasm.

For erection deflation in the middle of things, avoid getting upset about it. Stress and anxiety constrict the arteries, including the ones that carry blood into the penis. If you get upset about a wilting erection, it's likely to wilt even more. Instead, breathe deeply, ask for the kind of penile stroking or sucking that turns you on, and focus on a hot, juicy erotic fantasy. Taking these steps won't necessarily produce the fireworks you recall from your twenties, but they'll make sex noticeably more pleasurable for you.

Aches, Pains, Positions, and Props

Chances are, our bodies just don't do what they used to. But if we get creative, this doesn't have to be a major problem. Many people wrote me about ways to avoid aches and pains during sex. Here's what some of them had to say.

ZOSHI, AGE 68

I have arthritic knees and hands, so I can't take an upper position easily, and it can be a challenge to keep up manual stimulation of my partner if the arthritis is kicking in. He has his own aches and pains, so a sense of humor is our most valuable asset. Finding positions that will allow us to both be comfortable can be tricky, but we found a scissors position on our sides that works. Oral sex is facilitated with the use of a pillow under my hips, or he kneels on a pillow at the bedside. The 69 position is more difficult, so we take turns. I can hold myself on my side with my arm or elbow for some time, with him on his back for me to reciprocate.

KATH, AGE 68

There is little information available about sex following a total hip replacement. My doctor blushed and cringed when I mentioned the subject. After the operation, I observed eight weeks of prescribed abstinence. The missionary position is an ideal starter position for safe postoperative sex, as long as the leg isn't drawn up too far. As time goes on, unless you're into extreme acrobatics, almost any position is fine. A day will come when you no longer even think about your hip.

CHLOE, AGE 70

How do we have sex comfortably with our aging bodies—with arthritis, stiffness, and circulation problems? Are there any chairs, or other furniture, that will enhance our ability to have sex more easily? Someone needs to design something so the partners can be more comfortable when performing these acts.

Joan Responds

Actually, Chloe, "sex furniture" has been designed already for our comfort. Robert and I used the Liberator Wedge—a perfectly shaped, firm, triangular pillow designed for sex (though it also made a good back support for reading in bed, we discovered). At some of my workshops, I set aside embarrassment to demonstrate how I could lie on my back, with my hips elevated by the Wedge. This was not only good for my back, but also for Robert's, because he didn't have to curve over. Liberator makes other pillow forms that suit whatever position you might enjoy, with support where you need it. The wedge is available from many of the sex shops I recommend at www .NakedAtOurAge.com.

We need more than jar openers, reading glasses, and non-slip rugs at our age. The more we talk out loud about senior sex, the more likely inventive folks will see an opportunity to provide what we need!

A Healthy Older Woman Is a Sexy Older Woman

Older people—especially healthy ones, and especially men—are enjoying sex, according to a study published in the *British Medical Journal* in March 2010.[1] When the study came out, the media were all over it, sometimes with shudders and distaste *(Wrinkly people enjoying sex? Eeewww.)*; sometimes with a health message

(Eating right and exercising leads to good sex, even when you're old.); and sometimes with an emphasis on the disparity between genders *(Old men like it; old women don't . . . huh!)*.

After the study came out, sex educator Ellen Barnard wrote me in frustration about the focus on the gender disparity in this study, especially because no one was looking into the *reasons* why older women aren't enjoying sex more and what they can do about it. Here's what she had to say.

An Expert Responds

ELLEN BARNARD, MSSW

According to this study in the British Medical Journal, older women stop having and enjoying sex sooner in their lives than men do. That's because the medical community has no idea how to help women maintain their sexual health and pleasure after menopause without the use of potentially dangerous hormones. The truth is, there are simple answers.

- Healthy women enjoy good sex much longer than those in poor health. Live a "good-sex lifestyle," which includes daily exercise and a healthy diet—one that's full of fruits, veggies, nuts, whole grains, and healthy fats. Stay away from white sugars and flours, maintain a low-to-moderate alcohol intake, and take daily doses of chocolate, omega-3 oils, and vitamin D.

- During and after menopause, care for your vagina. Moisturize it daily or more often with a good moisturizing lubricant (no glycerin), and massage the inner walls two to four times per week for five to ten minutes, with either a well-made vibrator or a partner's fingers or penis. For more details, see our Vaginal Renewal program (http://bit.ly/vrprogarticle).

- Have at least one orgasm per week, with yourself or a partner—it doesn't matter. Keep those nerves functioning properly, and remind them what pleasure feels like. If it's hard to have orgasms, use a vibrator.

- Get enough sleep, keep your stress under control, and keep a positive outlook. Your body will thank you for it, and your mind will be able to enjoy sex without distraction.

- Think sexy thoughts, often. Fantasize, reminisce, create erotic stories in your head or on paper, talk about sex, plan for sex, and make it a priority. Nurture your sex life, and it will love you back for many years to come.

Lubricants: Bringing Back the Joy of Friction

It's a fact that most women don't lubricate as much after menopause, and often not sufficiently for sexual comfort and pleasure. That's why the universe invented lubricants. With them, our bodies can become as juicy as our minds.

Many women wrote to me with comments or questions about lubricants. Here's what they had to say.

KATHLEEN, AGE 54

At forty-five, I broke up with the man I thought I would be with forever. I couldn't feel anything with anyone—physical or otherwise—for several years. I tried to have sex, thinking it might defrost my heart, but I physically couldn't complete the act. That's when I first experienced vaginal dryness.

The first man I tried to have sex with told me he had been in love with me for years. We had a lovely time with foreplay, and he made me feel very special and attractive. When he tried to enter me, I was too dry. I was embarrassed, and the next few moments were awkward and painful. I finally gave up, telling him he was simply too big since I had not had sex in many months. I gave him a wonderful blowjob. (I'm really good at that, and I enjoy it!) He continued to pursue me, but I was so put off by my first-time failure that I couldn't bring myself to try it again.

I was still in a sad, frozen place when I met Bob, a stonemason. I stopped to admire his work, and we started talking every day. After our first real date, we parked in the driveway. Like teenagers, we wrestled and struggled, and I felt like a beautiful, desirable woman again. A pent-up dam of sexual feeling washed over me. It was such a relief to feel like a whole woman again. It unlocked a door I thought was locked to me forever.

Now, knowing I may be dry, I use internal lubricants a couple of days before a date with my partner, and I use lubricants during sex. I am also using different sized vibrators to reintroduce that part of my anatomy to penetration. Sounds clinical here, but it's very satisfying. I continue to see Bob, and I still enjoy sex and all that goes with it!

CHARMMI, AGE 72

The lining of a seventy-two-year-old is much different from that of a twenty-seven-year-old. Do I request a sex partner to apply lubricant to his penis, or would he get pleasure from inserting it into my vagina, or do I do it behind closed doors?

Joan Responds

Charmmi, a lack of lubrication isn't a shortcoming that you have to hide. Make lubricant part of the love play. Keep the bottle in plain sight and easy reach. It's arousing to both partners to apply lube to our own and each other's genitals with slow, silky strokes.

When Robert and I made love, this was one of our favorite parts. Even the act of getting the lubricant from the drawer was an erotic signal. When it was time to apply it, we would look into each other's eyes, then kiss for a long time, as we readied each other for intimate touch by transferring the lubricant from our hands to the other's waiting genitals with loving caresses.

ASHLEY, AGE 75

About five years ago, I realized that I was not lubricating as much as I had previously. K-Y or other over-the-counter lubricant didn't do the job, and I was finding intercourse painful. My gynecologist had never asked me about sex in any way—which I think was a failing on her part. A close friend told me she had been using Vagifem (estradiol vaginal tablets, an estrogen product). When I went for my gynecological checkup after about a year's use, the doctor said, "You have a very youthful vagina. I rarely see a vagina like yours in a woman over seventy."

Choosing Your Lube

BY MEGAN ANDELLOUX

Decreased vaginal lubrication often is a result of hormonal changes in a woman's body or medications. Even if your vagina is lubricating, your natural lubrication may not find its way to the clitoris. Lubrication on the clitoris can result in a woman experiencing more sexual satisfaction and easier orgasm. Applying lubricant is also important for anal play, because the anus/rectum does not create its own lube.

Decide what type of play you plan to have before choosing your lube. Certain lubricants work better for certain types of sex. If you are confused, ask before buying.

Petroleum-based lubricants, such as mineral oil and Vaseline, are not good internally, as they take a while to clear out of the system. They irritate vulvas, destroy condoms, and stain fabric. They're great for external male masturbation, though—cheap and easily accessible.

Natural oil-based lubricants—such as vegetable, corn, avocado, peanut, and olive oils—are safe to go inside the vagina. The body can clear out natural oils. However, they destroy condoms and stain fabric. They're fine for genital massages, safe to eat, cheap, and easily accessible.

Water-based lubricants with synthetic glycerin—such as Astroglide, KY Liquid/Jelly, Embrace, Replens and Liquibeads (suppositories for dry vaginal walls)—are commonly sold in supermarkets and drugstores. Glycerin produces a slightly sweet taste. However, these lubes dry out quickly and are often sticky or tacky. Plus, synthetic glycerin can be an open

➤

invitation for yeast infections. They're cheap, easy to find, safe with latex condoms, and do not stain fabric.

Water-based lubricants without synthetic glycerin—such as Maximus, Liquid Silk, Slippery Stuff, O'My, Sliquid, Sensua Organics, and Probe—do not trigger yeast infections. They last longer than lubricants with glycerin, can reduce irritation to the genitals, do not stain fabric, and are safe with latex condoms. These lubes can have a bitter taste due to the absence of glycerin. Saliva, an always accessible, water-based lubricant, tends to dry up more quickly than most commercial lubricants.

Silicone lubricants—such as Eros, Wet Platinum, ID Millennium, and Pink—last the longest of all lubricants and are safe to use with condoms. These lubes are more expensive but are ideal for sensitive genitals. They stay on underwater, are odorless and tasteless, and last three times as long as water-based lubricants. Silicone lubricants should not be used with silicone or cyberskin sex toys. Note that they are extremely flammable—do not use them with candles nearby.

Buyers beware: Do not use any lubricant with lidocaine or benzocaine, which are designed to reduce discomfort through numbing. These ingredients dull pain, which is the body's natural defense mechanism to alert you that something is possibly tearing in your body.

Making Time for Sex

Just because some of us are retired doesn't mean we're not still busy. Sometimes we have to make a special point of making time for sex, or it doesn't happen.

I always suggest scheduling "sex dates" at my sex-and-aging workshops, and attendees balk at first. "Sex should be spontaneous," they say. "It's not sexy if we schedule it."

Give it a chance. You may find that scheduling sex encourages you to think about it all day, anticipate what you'll do, and rev up your arousal.

Robert and I made special "sex dates," where we designated several hours of love time two afternoons a week. We drew hearts in our calendars to mark these dates. Scheduling several hours gave us time to first dance together, or to go for a walk and talk over the day, feeling our closeness, our footsteps, and our thoughts in rhythm with each other. We'd have the best sex after an hour of doing something physical together that wasn't sexual but that got us in touch with our own bodies and each other's. We coupled this activity with talking together, and our discussions were sometimes playful, sometimes profound. This too was making love.

By the time we were ready to go to bed, we were in sync. We'd send each other intimate signals: Starting a vibrator humming when the other was in the shower meant, "Join me, I'm getting ready for you." Wearing silk underwear meant, "Touch me slowly." Lighting candles meant, "I feel romantic—kiss me sweetly for a while." If it was afternoon, lighting candles also meant, "We'll still be in bed after dark."

Becoming Lovers Again

BY CHIP AUGUST

Many couples in their fifties and sixties are struggling with unsatisfactory sex lives. As young, sexually active adults, we take for granted that feelings of arousal will be accompanied by the swelling of genital tissues; erections of nipples, clitoris, and penis; and lubrication. In our minds we link these physical experiences to the idea of arousal.

Later in life, when erections and lubrication are less certain, we falsely assume that it is the end of sexuality. It's as if we have forgotten all the other emotions and sensations associated with arousal—how hot it once was to hold hands, to kiss, to talk nonsense for hours, to dance, to finish each other's sentences.

Becoming lovers again means behaving as lovers do. When we are in "new relationship energy," we gaze into each other's eyes, kiss, phone, and email. We send cute cards, buy flowers, go out to dinner, and take long walks. We make time just for us.

As long-term couples, we often curtail these behaviors. If we spent as little time and attention working at our jobs as we spend on our relationship, most of us would be unemployed. Relationships take time. Make dates. Park by the lake or the overlook, and neck like you were seventeen again. Get naked together and just hold each other and talk. If you get physically aroused, great! If not, notice how sweet it feels just to hold each other close.

Our biggest erogenous zone is between our ears—our minds. Sex isn't just a piece of skin wiggling around in some other skin. Sex is about intimate connection and shared

➤

> vulnerability. Sex is stroking each other from head to toe, eye-gazing, shared laughter, and shared thoughts. Sex is kissing, hugging, and dancing. Sex is lying naked in each other's arms, listening to our hearts beating.

HARRY, AGE 87

My wife and I married in our early twenties. We went through courtship, marriage, open marriage, raising a family, remote marriage, and now courtship all over again. We stayed together for the sake of the kids years ago, and now it is starting to pay off.

My wife and I stopped having sex after she had a complete hysterectomy at forty. She said she didn't feel like a woman any longer. I sought and found casual sex elsewhere. I left her alone far too much.

Now my wife and I have patched up our marriage, and I am trying to help her enjoy sex. She always was sexually passive. Now that she is older, she has become affectionate and more interested in sex.

What was exciting then is irritating now, so I proceed very slowly. She tells me that touching her bare breasts does not arouse her as it used to. She allows me to touch her breasts as long as I don't spend too much time on her nipples, since that irritates her. Kissing and holding her close arouses her. My wife asked me a little while ago to express my love by using endearments when talking to her.

I have the inhibitions of her youth to contend with. I mentioned the words "oral sex" and she was disgusted. It was something her generation of women seldom indulged in. I found this also applied to deep kissing, which I find erotic, because the tongue is like a penis as it seeks entrance. Masturbation is another subject we never discuss. I don't know how to close this big gap, or if I should maybe just accept "no."

Nature leaves an older man with all his sexual feelings, even if erection doesn't come easy any more. Getting an erection at my age requires the cooperation of my wife, and I am still working on getting her to touch my penis.

The key words are "patient" and "gentle" when it comes to lovemaking at eighty-plus. It takes endearments, kissing, and affection, as well as time together talking over the past. Pillow talk is important, as is going through our memories about when we met and how we got to know each other. It was enough then to lead to intimacy, and it still is.

Sex comes in many forms, I am finding out. Now, I find it is a matter of wooing her all over again.

2

Reviving Desire

I WANT MY SWEET tooth back!" a beautiful gray-haired woman announced in my workshop. She described how sexually juicy she used to be, both emotionally and physically: always ready for sex, driven by the urge she welcomed and enjoyed. Now, although she has sex, it never feels urgent. She misses that driving desire.

It makes sense that we don't have that driving urge. We're no longer biologically driven to reproduce. Our "I must have sex *now*" hormones have receded, and we desire sex for other reasons: to be touched, to enjoy our arousal and orgasm, to bond with our partner, to release stress, to have fun, to feel whole and fully alive. Emotional and physiological needs abound, but they're not the biological force that we experienced during our fertile years.

Maybe we're not spontaneously turned on by a thought, a kiss, or the shedding of underwear. But we can learn ways to nurture our sexual selves. Changes in our desire and arousal pattern are normal, and though they're disconcerting, they don't have to impact our relationship negatively or make us retreat from sex. We may need to get to know our changing bodies and brains all over again, but as long as we realize that this isn't a lack or a loss, we can enjoy the journey.

The experts in this chapter offer food for thought and practical tips to put the sizzle back into your sex life.

"Is It My Body or My Brain?"

Arousal and desire used to be united, thanks to our hormones. Now they may operate separately. Are you not feeling desire—that is, does sex not interest or appeal to you anymore? Or are the changes in arousal and sensation just making it more challenging to get physically stimulated enough to feel sexual pleasure?

If you *are* interested, but you arouse slowly, that's common. As we get older, the flow of blood to our genitals and our nerves' response to sexual stimulation both slow down. To help counteract this, you can keep yourself as healthy as possible with a nutritious diet and regular exercise, work on communication with your partner, reduce the stress in your life, and take plenty of time for sexual pleasure. Stay in the habit of regular orgasms—one or more a week—whether you're partnered or solo. The more you nurture your sexual responses, the better they'll keep working.

Sometimes it's hard to figure out whether your drop in libido is due to a decrease in desire or physiological changes affecting arousal and sensation. It's important to take note, especially when changes come on suddenly. Annie's shocking story illustrates the most important piece of advice in this whole book: *If you experience any sudden or extreme changes in how your body feels or responds, get thee to a doctor.* Get checked out. You'll hear this advice over and over again in this book, because it's that important.

ANNIE, AGE 75

How in the world could I not want sex with the love of my life? How could I still remember the thrills, fun, and joy of our sex, and yet not be interested? I wish I'd had an expert to talk to about this, because it could have saved my twelve-year relationship.

My partner was fifteen years younger than I was. I loved sleeping with her and holding her, but for no reason I could understand, my interest in sex stopped. The sex we used to share was of no interest to me. We went to a gynecologist, but all she did was give me some cream to put on my clit, and that was it. Obviously, that didn't resolve the problem.

My partner began to think I didn't love her, or that I was getting too old for sex. Before long she walked out the door with a friend of ours. That was eleven years ago, and I've not seen her since.

Two months after she left, I had a heart attack. My lack of libido had a cause, after all—it turned out to be heart disease!

This is what I learned about desire changing: If partners love each other and it happens to one, love them more and help them find a doctor! Loss of desire can very well be a symptom of an illness. Six months after my partner left, I had two stents put in my heart vessels, which were 100 percent closed. I went through this terror without the love of my life. She was the one person I wanted at my side, but she was two thousand miles away with her new love.

I recently had a quadruple bypass surgery, and who did I want by my side? You guessed it. But after eleven years, I have no idea where she is.

I asked Myrtle Wilhite, MD, to explain the importance of how heart disease and lack of arousal are related in women, as well as men.

Sudden Loss of Arousal: Get Checked Out

BY MYRTLE WILHITE, MD, MS

If you're experiencing sudden changes in the experience of arousal or sensation, ask your doctor to evaluate you for heart disease, type 2 diabetes, and high blood pressure. There is clear evidence in the medical literature that erectile dysfunction precedes active symptoms of heart disease by four to five years. So erectile dysfunction in men, and its corollary of loss of arousal and sensation in women, are clear signals that there is something wrong with blood flow in the body.

Women have to be persistent in asking for evaluation for heart disease, as the signs and symptoms in women are not yet well understood. Insist on tests—even if they are expensive—if you are experiencing any symptoms that make you wonder about your body's ability to move blood into (and out of) all the small blood vessels successfully.

Get yearly checks of your bodily inflammation (the test is called highly sensitive C-reactive protein, or hs-CRP), and if this level is high, that's another warning sign. Other warning signs include metabolic syndrome (which precedes type 2 diabetes), smoking, a lack of daily exercise, and a diet high in saturated fats and sugars and low in whole foods, fruits, and vegetables.

If your doctor isn't willing to help with these preventive measures, get a new doctor. Anyone who tells you that it's in your head or that all you need is a vibrator is not paying good attention to what may be underlying your symptoms.

Note: For more about the "good sex lifestyle," see Ellen Barnard's advice in Chapter 1.

JILL, AGE 53

Is there a physiological reason why I have no interest in sex? Is there a way to tell if my long-term use of Prozac will affect me for the rest of my life? I took it for sixteen years and only got off of it two months ago. When I first started taking it—while in a very passionate relationship—I could tell a big difference in my sexual response.

I'm gay. (In my opinion, "lesbian" is a term for people who live in Greece.) I haven't felt sexual since age forty-eight or so—although who can say whether the change is age-related, health-related, emotional, or situational.

Before that, I had a very intense sexual and emotional relationship with a woman who was fifteen years older. My response to her was passionate and satisfying. However, she started to withdraw from me sexually. I was very frustrated. She left me four years ago, and I haven't had those kinds of feelings for anyone since.

Nothing turns me on. Nothing about me looks or feels sexy. Sex toys disgust me. I think if you have to use something, why bother? I do get lonely. I live in an area where there are few, if any, single gay women.

I wonder if women are really that interested in sex. It's a part of life, but as one gets older and has already had a good sex life earlier, other things become important. I think the emphasis should be on fulfilling emotional needs.

The way that I have gone about meeting women and getting into relationships in the past was a result of the spark of sexual chemistry. Now that this is not a conscious part of my life, how do I go about seeking out suitable partners, for companionship, or whatever?

An Expert Responds

ELLEN BARNARD, MSSW

Jill, your reason for having no interest in sex is probably not physiological, although you may have a harder time recognizing sexual arousal and interest in your body. That can make you feel like your body is just not sexual any longer.

Orgasmic delay and difficulty are the primary sexual side effects of Prozac, but the long-term use of Prozac should not affect you for the rest of your life. Generally, the system that is affected by Prozac will be back to normal within a year of stopping the medication. You should find that your ability to have orgasms will improve over the next ten months, as long as you are in good health and are keeping your sexual system in good condition by exercising it regularly. (That is, by having orgasms.)

When you question whether the change is age-related, health-related, emotional, or situational, you make a good point. Desire is complex, and all the things you mentioned can affect how sexual you feel.

It sounds like losing your last relationship was difficult for you. Have you done some exploration to find out how the loss of this relationship may be affecting your self-image? You may have internalized feelings about the breakup that are making you feeling undesirable or unlovable—which may in turn make you feel unsexual. That might be a good place to start with a counselor.

Sex toys have been around for thousands of years for a reason: They are useful tools for helping us enjoy the sensations of sexual pleasure. A good, practical sex toy would help you exercise your sexual-arousal system in a way that would keep it primed and responsive.

The sexual parts of us need to be activated regularly to work well and to respond to sexual thoughts in a noticeable way—particularly as we get older. The longer you are out of practice with enjoying stimulation, arousal, and orgasm, the slower your body responds, and the more difficult it is to get turned on. Whether you choose to self-stimulate using your own hands or a tool designed for the job doesn't matter, but it is important to nurture your sexual self.

Many older women are interested in sex—if they have a strong sense of connection to that part of themselves, and if they continue to encourage themselves to stay sexual.

If you want a companion, you'll want to seek out women who share similar interests and life goals with you. You may or may not feel a "spark," but you're likely to have a good friend. Some women are content with that sort of a connection, and you'll want to be clear from the outset about whether you're seeking a friend, companion, or lover.

The other possibility is that you start making sex and the connection to your sexual self a conscious part of your life. Most midlife women find that they have to be more conscious about choosing to become aroused and then following that arousal on to further pleasure. They need to deliberately fantasize, read erotica, watch erotic scenes, and generally be more proactive about creating a space for sex in their lives. Once you start being consciously sexual, you'll find it happens more often, more easily, and more rewardingly.

Note: For more about vibrators and how they can rev up your sexual responsiveness, see Chapter 3.

Sex and Emotions

BY CAROL QUEEN, PHD

Whether it's your relationship with your partner, stress, or feelings about your changing body, your emotional life affects your sexual interest and response.

The quality of a woman's relationship often makes itself felt in her enjoyment of sex with her partner. Unaddressed frustration, anger, resentment, and other so-called "negative" emotions can, over time, undermine a woman's sexual desire with her partner. Sometimes this is enough to turn her off sex in general. Other times it raises her willingness to get sexual satisfaction elsewhere.

Stress and worry affect sexual desire. Any kind of life crisis—from the death of a pet to a job loss—can affect your libido, as can body image.

Having a male partner who isn't getting erections anymore is not a reason to stop having sex, nor should it be a reason for relationship problems. In reality, of course, it very often does cause such problems, either because a woman assumes her partner's lack of erection is a comment on his level of interest, or because a man completely associates an erection with sexual pleasure that he thinks it's all over and withdraws from intimate contact. This is an issue that can really affect a couple, but does not need to spell the end of their sex life at all.

In the Mood

If you wish you were in the mood for sex but you're not, pretend you are. If you let yourself get aroused physically, it's likely that the mood will follow. It often works, and it's one important key to improving your sexual relationship if you don't have the urge you used to.

Please don't misunderstand me—I am not suggesting you give in to pressure to have sex when you don't want to, or when it's painful or distasteful, or when the relationship is unhealthy. I'm also not suggesting you should fake orgasms or otherwise be dishonest with your partner (see the next section). I am suggesting that if you're in a loving relationship, you give your sexy feelings a chance to surface by understanding that, at our age, arousal often follows action, rather than the other way around.

In order to desire it, do it—and the desire will kick in once you become physiologically aroused. And the more you have pleasurable sex, the more you'll want to have it. Cool how that works!

Maybe it's as simple as making love during your high-energy time of day instead of at nighttime or after a meal, when your blood is going to your digestive system rather than to your genitals. Robert and I found a huge jump in arousal and desire when we made love in the daytime rather than at night. We would schedule sex dates for either mid-morning or mid-afternoon, the times that worked best for us.

Another thing we did to get in the mood was kiss. Just kiss. We kissed quietly without disconnecting, paying attention to each other's breath. It slowed us down, quieted our minds, and made us aware of each other and of our own pleasure centers. Our breathing got in sync, and as we continued to kiss, something magical happened. We felt we were melting into each other, one body, one breath. Our skin started tingling, our pleasure receptors came alive. We felt each other shudder with excitement, and we were making love.

Women: How to Get Going
When You Don't Feel the Urge

BY DIANA WILEY, PHD

Mismatched sexual desire is the Number One problem discussed in sex therapists' offices. Usually it is the woman with
lower desire. Conflicts develop when lovers have significantly
different sexual appetites.

Erotic feelings flow most easily when a woman feels confident, secure, and relaxed. Stress, fatigue, depression, grief, negative body image, and unresolved issues interfere with desire.
So do continuing arguments and feelings of anger.

What to do? *Just do it!* New research suggests that, for
more than half the population, sexual desire doesn't just happen. Desire may not precede arousal. Most women have to be
physically stimulated to feel desire. So women who think they
need to be in the mood to have sex, might in fact need to have
sex to be in the mood! In other words, *just do it!* Countless
clients have told me they didn't want to do their "just do it"
homework—but once they got into it, they really started to
enjoy themselves.

Using Mindfulness

Women's brains are designed to multitask. It comes from the
days of needing to hear a baby's cry no matter what else we
were doing—including making love. Even if our children have
left the nest decades ago, the tendency to focus on several
things simultaneously persists. This can interfere with our ability to enjoy sex and let everything else go.

➤

However, we can develop our ability to stay in sync with the body's responses. Pay attention to the senses: What do you see, smell, taste, hear? Imagine putting your wandering thoughts on a conveyor belt and watching them slowly roll away. Be in the moment. Keep your eyes, pores, and brain open. Surrender to your sensations, and stay "in the moment." A bonus: Orgasms are much more likely in such a state.

Mindfulness is especially necessary for the sensate focus exercises developed by the Masters and Johnson research team. You can relearn how to give pleasure through touching. Begin with simple caressing and sensual massage from head to toe, and move slowly toward more intimate erotic contact. Initially, do the exercises without moving toward intercourse; this will alleviate any performance anxiety. The entire body is an instrument available for tuning: ears, neck, small of the back, fingertips, toes.

Keeping It Playful

The most neglected sexual art these days is laughter, true mirth. The aphrodisiac of laughter can encourage and even prolong pleasure. And one way to generate spontaneous laughter is to use the element of surprise. If you've been Rebecca of Sunnybrook Farm for twenty years, you probably won't want to jump out of the closet wrapped in Saran Wrap and with a vibrator in each hand. But be inventive in your own unique way. Change the pattern, change the place, change your approach, change your response, change your style.

Incorporating Fantasy

Especially in the early stages of a relationship, the brain produces dopamine, the hormone of arousal. But dopamine needs novelty. To create this novelty, some people may need to create the illusion that they're with a stranger by using sexual fantasy. Rodney Dangerfield once described a time when he and his wife were trying to make love but nothing was happening. "What's the matter?" he asked. "Can't you think of anyone either?" Fantasy is a way of enriching a sexual relationship!

ZOSHI, AGE 68

It was a big shock to me that much of my libido was hormone-related. I thought my strong sexual appetite was me, not my hormones. I don't have as much sensation, as much arousal, or as easy orgasms, nor am I as driven to inappropriate behavior as I once was. It's definitely a loss on the one hand and a release on the other. Though the longer time it takes to orgasm can make me sore, and the range of activity that will get me there is considerably narrower, I've learned to operate with the subtler energies available to me now.

ADVICE FROM AN EXPERT

Lose the Mood

BY FRANCESCA GENTILLÉ

Don't worry about being in the mood or getting in the mood for sex. If you practice the "sacred sexuality essensuals," the mood will follow:

- breathe

- relax

- reconnect with the love of this person

- remember the good times

- let go of "have to," "should," and performance

- pet and praise your partner's body, using long, affectionate strokes, which release oxytocin, increasing blood flow and creating a feeling of well-being and bonding

After twenty minutes of breathing and petting, the genitals engorge, the brain waves change, and the arousal system is pumped. Your body and your partner's will awaken to their potentials for connection and arousal.

After the body awakens, start including the genitals. Our genitals love pets, pats, caresses, and adoration too. Be the No. 1 fan of your beloved's genitals.

I Can't Tell Him

It used to be so simple: When we got aroused, we experienced that delicious tingling and swelling in the genitals and we lubricated freely. Now arousal is more elusive. It may take longer, it may feel different, and it may take another kind of love play to coax our pleasure to the surface. Faking it with our partner will just keep us stuck and dissatisfied.

This is the time for honesty. I don't think faking it ever nurtures a relationship, especially not at our age.

Better to talk honestly; to discover together what you need to get aroused. Maybe it's a lot of love play before you get under the covers. Maybe bringing sex toys into your relationship would aid your arousal. Your partner would appreciate knowing the truth and join you in the journey to discovery of what turns you on.

TERRI, AGE 52

I am starting to lose my desire for sex. I have been dating a man in his early forties for about eight months now. He is very sexual, and although I enjoy making love with him, I just don't get excited as easily as he does. I don't want him to think he doesn't turn me on, so I pretend a lot. I can't tell him that I don't have the desire, because I'm afraid he'll either feel rejected or look for someone younger. I hate the way my body is betraying me, and I really want to enjoy sex, but I just can't tell him this. Any suggestions on how to rekindle my desire? I don't want to take hormones, because they scare me to death.

An Expert Responds

ELLEN BARNARD, MSSW

As we get older, blood flow to our genitals gets slower, and our nerve response to sexual stimulation also slows down. We may experience changes in arousal and sensation that make it take longer—and require more work—to get adequately aroused for pleasure. Here are some strategies for overcoming arousal difficulties and the problems they may cause in your relationship with your partner.

Become familiar with how arousal feels in your body now that you're lubricating less quickly and less noticeably. Most women rely on the obvious feeling of wetness and the fairly quick rush of swelling to tell them that they are turned on. But as we age, this happens more slowly and subtly. As a result, it can be harder to notice, so we may think we're not becoming aroused, even when we actually are.

Spend some time self-pleasuring, and pay attention to how your growing arousal feels. Where do you feel it? What works to make the sensation more noticeable and pleasurable? Does your arousal increase when you fantasize? If so, what images work best?

This inventory of "what works and how I can tell it's working" will be useful when it comes to sharing this knowledge with your partner.

Also, work on communicating with your partner about the changes that are happening in your body, and what these changes mean to your sexual relationship. While I know it's difficult, it's important to stop pretending and start sharing what you need and want to make sex great for both of you. We are all afraid of offending our partners, but the biggest compliment we can pay is to take the risk and share what's true and real in our hearts, so that we can enjoy the pleasure we want, together.

One way to start the conversation is to say something like, "You may have heard that women go through changes as we age. That's happening to me." You can then explain that it takes longer for you to be aroused, and that you want to be sure he knows that he does turn you on—it just takes longer and a little more work. Have a good lubricant available, and the two of you can work together to figure out how to make it fun and sexy to use it together.

Practice asking for what you need in a way your partner can hear it. Rather than saying "I'm just not enjoying sex with you," say, "I've noticed some things about my body and how it responds during sex that I want to share with you so we can both enjoy the best sex with each other."

Of course, you need to know what works for you, so explore on your own, using lubricant and maybe a vibrator. Then share what you have learned with your partner. A worthy partner will be glad to know what works for you and will want to join you in exploring new ways to make sure you enjoy sex.

Yes, We Do Look Sexy!

So we don't look like we did in our twenties, and we never will again. (Probably in our twenties, we didn't like the way we looked either!) But we are the youngest we'll ever be from now on, and if we see ourselves as sexy, we're more likely to feel sexy and to be sexy.

Here's a shortcut to seeing yourself as sexy—buy some pretty lingerie, and see how gorgeous you look in the mirror. I'm not kidding about the effect that can have on your self-image. Near my sixty-sixth birthday, I agreed to do a lingerie shoot with a photographer who wanted to capture the sexiness of real women with real bodies and faces. I couldn't believe how much fun it was, and how easily I slid from "Please don't photograph my belly!" to "I am sexy and gorgeous!"

We all have the right—and the ability—to feel that way about ourselves. No one can "make us" feel it. We have to create that feeling for ourselves.

JORDANA, AGE 55

What happened to my libido? I need some excitement infusion here! My husband and I have been together nineteen years. We are very affectionate—hugging, kissing, stroking, and snuggling—but there is little charge for me. Most of the time, I am not that interested until we get started, and then I get into the spirit. Despite this, my orgasms are much more intense now than in the past.

We have sex once or twice on weekends, and our sessions can last two or more hours. I really don't want any more than that, but my husband would like three to four times a week. We love to engage in oral sex, and for me, that is much more comfortable than penetration, even with adequate lube. My orgasms are intense that way.

I don't feel good about my body. I am about twenty pounds overweight, not in the best of shape, and I don't feel desirable. I like my face, hair, and feet, but anything in between is fair game for criticism. I know my husband doesn't find me sexy, although he enjoys having sex with me. I am less interested in engaging with him sexually since a lack of feeling sexy just doesn't get the arousal flowing.

His words and actions are a big part of the equation. My husband was never one for verbal foreplay. "What time do you want to have sex?" was his approach. I would like him to give me more verbal expressions of my attractiveness, and what he would like to do with me, well before we hit the sack. I need the "big buildup."

We've worked through this issue many times. It's gotten better, but I never felt desired, so I just turned it off within myself. That, coupled with hormonal changes and dryness, led to my lack of interest. I also think anger, depression, irritation, and frustration had a big part in lessening my desire.

My husband thinks about and desires sex constantly, and he has been disappointed by my lack of interest. I've explained to him that this has a lot to do with his actions and deeds. Sometimes his needs annoy me.

About five years ago, I took some striptease classes, and that really spiced things up for a while. But then we got back into a rut—with me feeling unattractive and with him not doing all that much to convince me otherwise—and things took a tumble. As challenging as sex has been for me of late, I still value it and want to nurture it.

Joan Responds

Jordana, other readers may envy you your two-hour lovemaking sessions, but that aside, it's clear you're unhappy. You don't feel good about yourself, your body, or your husband's libido.

Your story illustrates several issues that women our age are facing. You're carrying an extra twenty pounds, and you don't think you look attractive or desirable. All of this makes you feel far from sexy.

But rather than taking charge of your self-image by embarking on an exercise program and perhaps investing in lingerie that highlights your best assets, you want your partner to "make you" feel sexy and desirable. Feeling attractive and desirable can only come from within. We have to create those feelings ourselves.

This doesn't mean that your husband wouldn't benefit from learning communication skills to help you get in the mood—you're right to ask for that kind of verbal foreplay. But you also said that you see your husband's needs as "annoying," which must devastate your sexually eager husband. You say that you recognize that your feelings of "anger, depression, irritation, and frustration" have tamped down your desire.

Rather than blame your husband for your lack of desire, a couples' counselor could do wonders to help both of you break through your emotional and communication barriers to greater love, understanding, and sexual connection.

Act As If . . .

BY LAURIE MINTZ, PHD

Many of my clients are struggling with low sexual desire. Here are two straightforward, powerful techniques that have helped them.

Use self-affirmation. You may be reinforcing your belief that you're not sexy, desirable, or desirous by saying this to yourself. Counteract this by creating a sex-positive mantra that you repeat several times a day. Mantras work best when they are concise and tailormade to fit your own situation. If you are struggling with low sexual desire, your mantra might be something like "I love sex" or "I feel turned on." You can also post your mantra on your mirror or some other place where you're sure to see it daily.

While doing a mantra sounds simple, it's a powerful tool. We often come to believe what we repeatedly tell ourselves—so tell yourself what you want to believe.

We also become who we behave as—and this is the basis of the second technique: the "act as if" strategy, in which you act as if you already *are* who you want to be. If you don't feel sexy but wish you did, your task is to act as if you are the sexiest woman alive. If you don't feel desirous of sex but wish you did, you are to act as if you were hot for sex. As you go through your day, continually ask yourself, "How would someone who feels sexy act right now?" or "How would someone who was hot for sex act right now?" Then act according to your answer.

When I explain this technique to clients, a common concern is "Isn't that faking?" My reply is that faking is being

➤

deceitful—not being who you are. But this is quite different: It is stretching yourself to behave as the person you *want* to be. I have seen this simple technique result in great insights and behavioral changes.

Take a week and try it out: Act sexy or horny, or whatever it is you want and wish to be. I hope you will be as pleased as my clients have been.

Reaching Out to a Partner with Low Desire

Gauging from the questions and stories people send me, a lack of desire—even though everything still functions well—occurs much more with women than with men. I sometimes hear from men whose partners no longer desire sex as often, and they ask me what they can do. One way to open communication about this subject? Try giving your loved one this book, with a velvet bookmark marking this chapter.

JAKE, AGE 54

I've always been the high-libido or "needy" partner in my relationship with my wife, and I've had to deal with having my desires for a more adventurous and exciting (not to mention more frequent) sex life go largely unsatisfied, or one-sided at best. Over the years, I've had to become quite adept at the art of self-pleasuring.

I'm not really complaining. As a matter of fact, now that both of us are in our fifties, I have to say that our sex life is better than it has ever been—but not without having gone through a lot of friction and discord to get us to this point. We're still dealing with desire discrepancies that we'll never completely resolve, but at least we've managed to come to terms with it a lot better.

What can the high-libido partner do to raise the priority level of sex and intimacy when the other partner doesn't really see the need to concern herself with it at all? She seems to think that it'll either take care of itself or that it'll just go away altogether, and she'd be okay either way.

An Expert Responds

BARB DEPREE, MD

Jake, it's good that your sex life with your wife is better than ever, though the desire disparity sounds frustrating to you. For women, sex doesn't always begin with lust, but instead starts in our hearts and minds. The older we grow, the more this is true. We engage in our heads first, decide to have sex, and then, with enough mental and emotional stimulation, our genitals respond. For us, having sex is less an urge than a decision—one we can choose to make and then act upon. When we *decide* to say yes instead of no, when we *decide* to schedule sex instead of waiting for our body to spontaneously light on fire, when we *decide* to engage with methods that will put us in the mood rather than wait for romantic moments to magically happen, we're using our heads to keep sex in our relationships.

Deciding to be intimate unlocks the pleasure. And the more sex we decide to have, the more sex we will feel like having. That's the secret to regular bonding. For you and your wife, it may help you to decide, as a couple, to have sex on a certain regular basis.

Sex is important for other reasons too:

- It helps protect against heart attack and stroke, as does all exercise.

- The hormones released during sex decrease the risk of breast and prostate cancer.

- It bolsters the immune system.

- It helps us get to sleep.

- It can alleviate chronic pain, including migraines.

- An active sex life is closely correlated with overall quality of life.

- It can protect us against depression.

- It reduces stress and increases self-esteem.

- It stimulates feelings of affection, intimacy, and closeness with your partner.

Make sex a focus in your life as you get older, and know that you can engage in thoroughly satisfying sex without waiting around for desire. Just by using your head.

3

Sex Toys: Now More Than Ever

HERE'S WHERE OUR readers may divide into two camps: those who already use sex toys and those who don't. If you do, I hope you'll explore new ideas here. If you have never used one, or if the last time you used one was in your youth (and maybe then it was a cucumber), this chapter will open your eyes. Even if you came of age before vibrator use was commonplace, or even if you have convictions that they're unnatural, read this chapter thoroughly, trying to keep an open mind and a sense of adventure.

Bottom line: Whether you're single or partnered, sex toys can mean the difference between orgasm or not. It's sometimes that simple. As we get older, most of us find that sexual arousal takes longer and orgasm is harder to achieve due to age, illness, medications, or the emotions that interfere with sexual experience and/ or satisfaction. Both women and men of our age often need an extra assist. Sometimes a patient lover or extended time for self-love is all we need. But if arousal and orgasm are difficult, the right sex toy can send you into orbit in a way you thought had left your life forever. No kidding: Modern sex toys are that good. I speak from *plenty* of personal experience.

Getting Past Guilt, Fears, and Falsehoods

Women sometimes write to me about their reluctance or guilt about using vibrators, as if needing or wanting extra stimulation is an admission of a personal failing. Here's the way I see it: We don't object to putting moisturizer on our faces or a brace on our knee—so why not use vibrators to keep orgasms coming? It's far easier to reach an orgasm with the buzz from a clitoral vibrator than on our own. The extra boost of intensity may be just what our bodies require to fire. Orgasms are important for keeping the genitals healthy and the sexual responses coming. Think of it as physical therapy, if that makes it more palatable. Sex toys can be your bedtime buddy with a pet name—or just a tool for staying sexually vibrant.

Men also write to me about their concerns about vibrators. Some feel the need to inform me that nothing substitutes for the "real thing." Granted, but many women do not have a "real thing" relationship, and many who do still require a bit of buzzing to reach orgasm. Some men worry that using a vibrator will spoil a woman, who will then prefer it to a man. They insist that they've had relationships ruined by a vibrator.

Friends: Vibrators don't ruin relationships—they enhance them.

Myths and Facts about Vibrators

Despite the joy of toys, many women of our age who did not grow up with vibrators are reluctant to use them and have misconceptions. Here are some questions I've heard, with my comments.

> *"Doesn't using a vibrator decrease sensitivity over time so I won't have orgasms as easily?"*
> Actually, it's the opposite. As we age, we get less blood flow to the clitoris and vagina, and the vaginal walls get thinner. Most

of us need more arousal time *and* more time to reach orgasm after we're aroused. Vibrators enhance sensitivity by increasing blood flow to the genitals quickly and powerfully, and by directly stimulating the clitoris.

"My lover is worried that if I use a vibrator, I'll prefer it to him."
Not a chance. A vibrator may give you quicker orgasms, but it doesn't cuddle or kiss or laugh, and pillow talk with a vibrator is really boring. It's a dull companion—except when you need a sexual assist.

"My lover says I should reach orgasm "naturally" and not have to use a sex toy."
I hate those "shoulds." Explain to him where his penis contacts you during intercourse versus where your clitoris resides. And when he arouses you manually, which I hope he does, point out that he's less likely to get carpal tunnel syndrome from your long arousal time if he incorporates a vibrator in arousal play. It's not a choice between him or it. Make it a threesome: the two of you using the vibrator together.

"I had two friends who burned themselves with sex toys. Aren't they dangerous?"
The cheapest ones generally have no quality standards in materials or construction, and I don't recommend them. If your eyes widen at the price of the vibrators I recommend on my blog, consider that I only recommend safe products with medical-grade materials, careful construction, and the best design and function for our older bodies. You're paying for research and development and high-quality material that won't degrade, leach chemicals, break, overheat, or burn. That's also why I recommend shopping in woman-friendly sex

shops (brick-and-mortar or online) with an emphasis on health and education, like the ones I link to on my blog.

For more on the topic of safe sex-toy use, see the last section of this chapter.

Toys for Solo Sex

If you are single and your sex life is solo, sex toys can enhance this experience and make that elusive orgasm easier to achieve. Personally, as an unpartnered widow of two years, I would be in bad shape if I didn't use them. I'm serious. I know women of our age don't usually talk about this, but I think we should.

In fact, I've made my solo use of sex toys quite public. No, I don't whip out my favorite vibrator in coffee shops. I mean that I write about my sex-toy use now, sharing on my blog how well a particular product helps me achieve my goal. It was weird to do that at first. I never discussed vibrator use—not even with my best friends—until I went public in *Better Than I Ever Expected*. Not that I was ashamed—it just seemed profoundly personal to share how I aroused myself.

Ironically, it took being a widow to feel comfortable about writing about my personal vibrator use. I knew that I had the responsibility for my sexual health, and sex toys were my tools for keeping my sexuality alive.

I used toys from my past, and I started exploring new ones. I found, through my personal trial and error, that some worked really well for the special needs of an aging body and others didn't. Were the vibrations strong enough? Could it go long enough without overheating or becoming uncomfortable for arthritic wrists to hold? Was it made out of safe material? Could I figure out the controls without wearing reading glasses?

Often before I bought a toy, I read reviews online. They were very helpful (not to mention great fun to read), but they never addressed the questions an elder user might ask. So I started reviewing toys from a senior perspective on my blog. No one else was doing this. I became *the* "senior sex-toy reviewer" of the blogosphere. Retailers and manufacturers now send me sex toys in return for an honest review. I don't have to like what they send me, I just have to help my readers sort through the hundreds of available vibrators and accessories so that they can make informed choices.

"I love my job!" I often exclaim as I test a new toy and write my review. I hope you'll read my sex-toy reviews at www .NakedAtOurAge.com. Click the label SEX TOYS in the right-hand column. Your mileage may vary, but it's a good starting point to read reviews from a senior perspective.

Making sex toys part of a regular health practice (and I do see it that way) helps the blood circulate to the genitals and helps sexual thoughts circulate in our brains. And the right sex toy feels so darned good and leaves a smile on our happy, relaxed, glowing faces. Take it from Babs and Olivia.

BABS, AGE 50

I got my first vibrator only a few years ago, and I have discovered what orgasms really can be. Orgasms are much more intense and earth-shaking with a vibrator as stimulation.

OLIVIA, AGE 69

I've used a variety of sizes of penises (dildos) and some butter-fly kinds of things by myself. They helped keep my senses alive and ready, and gave me release when I needed it.

Sharing Your Toys

If you are coupled, you may find that using sex toys together or alone helps you redefine what turns you on, express and explore your sexuality, have orgasms, and keep your intimacy strong—even when life throws obstacles your way.

Robert and I often used vibrators to "warm up" in preparation for making love. I was always in the mood emotionally, but sometimes my body resisted joining my mind. So I would sometimes use a vibrator on "low" or a clitoral pump to get my body aroused a little before we started making love. Including sex toys to amp our excitement became as much a loving ritual as lighting candles and murmuring sweet words to each other.

Robert also learned to enjoy the stimulation of a vibrator. He would run it over his beautiful dancer's body, lingering where it felt best over silk underwear. "I'm getting ready for you," he would tell me. I would get excited watching his preparations and arousal. I squirmed in anticipation of touching him, and he teased me as well as himself when he made me wait.

Then we put the toys aside for the time being, pleasured each other with hands and mouth, and finally joined in the ultimate bonding. We made love for a long time, he holding back as I rode the rising waves. Then, when I was ready, he reached for our favorite vibrator for partner sex, the Eroscillator, and held it to my clitoris. The Eroscillator is particularly "partner-friendly" because its long wand and small (but potent!) vibrating attachment don't get in the way of partner intercourse. Without it, I couldn't have an orgasm during intercourse, period.

In the past few years, many more vibrator styles have emerged that are easy to use during intercourse—I don't want this to sound like a commercial for the Eroscillator. The sex toy reviews on my blog will introduce you to many you've never seen or heard of, with shapes that target the clitoris and slip easily between partners for use during intercourse as well as solo.

Jake also found that using a vibrator enhanced sex with his wife—in fact, it brought her to her first orgasm ever.

JAKE, AGE 54

I don't think my wife had ever experienced a true orgasm until after the birth of our second child in our midtwenties. We started experimenting, at my instigation, with using vibrators. They were called "marital aids" back then and had to be purchased from a local retailer, because there was no online shopping.

I saw her pleasure as an important ingredient of my own, and I was determined to do whatever it took to give her her first orgasmic experience. The lady in the "adult novelty" store recognized that I was a rank beginner, however enthusiastic. She knowingly steered me toward something far less intimidating for the first-time user than the ten-inch, flesh-colored, vibrating rubber dildo that I had been seriously considering.

She recommended a small, egg-shaped, plastic vibrator in mother-of-pearl with a small cord attached to a remote-control device to turn it on and to vary the intensity of vibration. It could be either held in place over the clitoris by hand or tucked between our bodies during face-to-face lovemaking.

It was perfect. My wife took to it on the first try and experienced her very first gut-wrenching, pussy-clenching orgasm with it. It gave her an explosive clitoral orgasm pretty much every time we used it.

Now my wife enjoys using vibrators of various sizes and shapes, holding them against her clitoris and labia. When my wife plays with a vibrator while we're making love, it increases the likelihood that she'll experience an orgasm. Plus, it takes the pressure off me to be the one solely responsible for her achieving it. It gives her control over her own pleasure.

I've tried using vibrators against my penis and nipples but I have better success using butt plugs and cock/ball rings, which I find erotic and both physically and mentally stimulating. I especially like the feel of wearing a vibrating butt plug that buzzes against my prostate gland. My orgasms that way are nothing short of incredible. I like to wear a cock ring when we engage in intercourse, because it helps me to maintain a harder erection for longer periods—I think of it as my "poor man's Viagra."

YOLA, AGE 51

Vibrators with a partner provide more fun and variety. And if he is done, he can use a vibrator on me without too much exertion on his part.

TOM, AGE 58

My wife and I have been together for thirty-eight years. I am taking medications for low testosterone and thyroid. My wife is taking antidepressants and blood-pressure medication. She had been on hormone replacement therapy (HRT) for ten years or so, so she thought it best to get off of it because of the cancer risk. Because of this combination of factors, my wife became unable to have orgasms, and with little lubrication, sex was often painful. Our sex life seemed to be drying up.

We decided to work on making it better. We started taking more time in our lovemaking and using lubricant, and that worked much better for us. I bought *Better Than I Ever Expected,* and it has been very helpful.

Unfortunately, no amount of foreplay or oral or manual stimulation was able to bring about an orgasm in my wife. This was really frustrating to me as well as to her, because our love-making felt one-sided. In the past, I knew her body and her response, and I could bring about orgasms by a combination of oral and manual massaging.

After reading *Better Than I Ever Expected*, we bought an Eroscillator. We had never experimented with sex toys. What a difference! The first time we tried it, we spent some time together getting warmed up, and I used the soft fingertip attachment on my wife. She had her first orgasm in years, and she cried in my arms afterward. This has made a huge difference in our lovemaking. My wife now has strong orgasms. I love being sure that I can please her.

We have learned that timing can be a factor. Because her blood-pressure medication appears to interfere with orgasms, we try to plan around it. First thing in the morning is great, because we have plenty of energy, and it has been at least twelve hours since she took her medication. I may take a Levitra before I go to bed so that it is still in effect in the morning. It would be great to be totally spontaneous, but the payoff for planning makes up for the lack of spontaneity. The Internet has been a great way to get information, and it is very easy to discretely purchase lubricants, massage oils, and sex toys that I might not find otherwise.

Choosing Lube for Your Toy

Now that most of us are not lubricating enough for partner sex, solo sex, or vibrator sex, using a lubricant is important.

But check to see what your vibrator is made of when choosing your lube. A silicone lubricant is nice and slick and works fine with condoms and most toy materials. However, manufacturers of silicone toys recommend a water-based lubricant, because a silicone lubricant may soften a silicone toy, or even ruin a soft, stretchy toy. A silicone cock ring, for example, will soften and then break when used with silicone lubricant, and dildos and plugs made of soft silicone will degrade, lose their shape, and possibly tear. If you love the slickness of silicone lube, you can always put a condom on your silicone vibrator to protect it.

Note: See Chapter 1 for more on lubricants.

Toys for Guys

Sex toys aren't just for women. They can be wonderful pleasure assists for men too, especially men our age. Charlie Glickman, who knows toys and the needs they fill, explains.

ADVICE FROM AN EXPERT

Sex Toys for Older Men

BY CHARLIE GLICKMAN, PHD

Although some folks have the idea that sex toys are just for women, it's great when men let go of that and discover their own sex-toy options.

I often hear from older men, "Can a cock ring make my erection harder?" The answer is "Sort of." Cock rings work by trapping blood in the penis, so they sometimes make your erection firmer or a bit larger while you wear it. Many men like the squeezing sensation that cock rings provide, and they can make orgasms more intense. Some men find that rings make them take longer to orgasm, and others find that the extra sensations make it happen sooner. So you'll need to experiment.

➤

Cock rings can be worn during solo sex or with a partner. If you want to use it during penetrative sex, move the snaps to the side so they don't irritate your partner. With some medical conditions that cause erection difficulties, cock rings can actually cause damage, so please get checked out by a sex-positive doctor first.

Sleeves are another great way to explore different ways to play on your own or with a partner. If you tried one years ago and were disappointed, know that the technology has improved a lot. Some are prelubricated and disposable (great for traveling); others are high-tech, with inner workings designed for maximum pleasure. There are easy-to-clean silicone models, and less-expensive elastomer versions. Using a sleeve with a partner is a great way to add a little fun, especially when health issues or other concerns limit the kinds of sex you can do. Plus, it can be lots of fun for partners to watch you pleasure yourself.

Let's not forget how much fun prostate play can be! While some men have concerns about anal play, I always point out that where your nerve endings are has nothing to do with sexual orientation. Lots of guys have discovered that prostate massage feels great and can even help reduce the size of an enlarged prostate. Prostate toys like the Aneros, the Naughty Boy, and the ProTouch are popular with men.

Men's sex toys open up plenty of new possibilities for you to experience pleasure, so don't hold yourself back. You may be surprised at how much you enjoy them.

Speaking of Safety

A male reader wrote me:

> *I got an email that advertised a vibrating dildo called "the jack rabbit." My wife and I have been married over twenty-five years. I think it may be the kind of gift she'd enjoy. According to a testimonial in the ad, one customer uses it four times a day! It makes me feel as though my wife, who I love, is getting short changed. I want her to come three or four times a day if she has that potential, because I love her, and I want her to feel good even when my penis is not up to the job. Do you think she'd be offended if I get her one in a pretty box with a nice card?*

Oh, where to start? Never, never base a purchase—of anything, not just a sex toy—on an email ad. For one thing, you might be responding to a scammer who wants to know your email address is live and to get your credit card—he or she might not even have a product for sale. Always buy from reputable retailers, whether online or in your neighborhood. And reputable retailers don't spam your email inbox.

Second, who says this product will give your partner three or four orgasms a day? Oh, that's right—the *ad* says "someone" said that. The ad can say anything it wants. I could claim that reading two pages of this book gave Ima Liar, from Nowhere, USA, four orgasms. And although it would be untrue and unethical, there's no law against my sending an email with that testimonial. Don't believe anything you read in an unsolicited email from a stranger. If email claims were true, I'd have a rock-hard-all-night-long, power-drill tool—I get at least three emails a day promising me that.

Even if this product is real, and even if the seller is promoting it because it's the best sex toy since the Hitachi Magic Wand (women, stop cheering—it's loud in here), that doesn't mean it's the right one for your partner. I love vibrators, but I'd find it creepy if a partner decided to pick out one for me instead of asking me what I wanted. I'm the only one who knows what I'd like, so I'd prefer to pick it out myself. I'd guess that's true for your lady love too.

Another option is to choose something that you think she'd like, then print out a picture of it to show her before ordering. The surprise might be spoiled, but I think you'd gain more points by letting her make her own choice.

ADVICE FROM AN EXPERT

Avoid These!
Unsafe Products and Practices

BY VIOLET BLUE

Sex toys are an awesome gateway to an incredible sex life. These silly, bizarre things can lead to hours of orgasmic exploration, self-discovery, sexual self-reliance, and even deeper intimacy between couples—or a hilarious comedy of errors, depending.

But not everything mass-marketed for sex is safe to use. It's always "buyer beware" when purchasing a sex toy, and you should be prepared with knowledge about the products.

As a start, *avoid the following:*

- Nonoxynol-9: Condoms and lubricants with this agent can remove skin—really! It is supposed to kill HIV, but it can cause cervical abrasions and can strip away rectal lining.

➤

- Numbing lubricants and desensitizing creams: If something you're doing hurts, you want to know it and back off. Otherwise, injury or infection can occur. When you can't feel pain, you are getting injured, period.

- Sugar/glycerin/glycerol: Any lubricants with sugar, colorings, and flavors should be avoided. Glycerin/glycerol is a sugar. Sugar feeds yeast, causing vaginal irritation. (That also means no whipped cream or chocolate as "dessert" during oral sex—keep sex and food separate!)

- "Novelty" sex toys: Sex toys labeled "for novelty use only" are cheaply made, tend to break easily, and may be made with noxious materials that you don't want inside your body. Stick to sex toys from the growing number of high-quality sex-toy companies in the United States, United Kingdom, and Sweden who do not market their toys as novelties, and who prize sexual health and pleasure as the key building blocks of their businesses and their products.

- Going from back to front: Never go from anus to vagina with body parts or sex toys. Even if you're squeaky clean from the shower, internal fecal bacteria can transfer. If you like anal stimulation with a sex toy, cover it with a condom.

4

Together yet Alone:
Is This My Marriage?

M ANY PEOPLE HAVE told me they are stuck in sexually and emotionally frustrating relationships. Some of them love their partners and want to work it out. Others have given up and are ready to leave.

You'll find this chapter more therapist-intensive than others, because I wanted not only to help the people who described their relationship crisis to me, but also to give you glimpses into how *you* might benefit from counseling if you're not resolving the sexual and emotional setbacks in your relationship. As a result, you might feel like you're eavesdropping on the beginnings of several therapy sessions.

No Sex, No Satisfaction

When one spouse drops out of the sexual partnership, the other spouse may feel bewildered and frustrated. Once the couple is out of the habit of being sexual together, it's difficult to get back in—especially when the nonsexual spouse won't talk about it. Jenny's story illustrates this.

JENNY, AGE 58

My husband is the perfect person for me, except that we have no sex. We have had sex only five times in five years of knowing each other. Is that crazy or what?

My husband, sixty-one years old, is my buddy and good friend whom I love—but he is not my lover. He is sexually dysfunctional due to blood-pressure pills. Viagra works well, but we are now stuck in "no sex mode." There always seems to be some reason we don't get together sexually. We go about our days accepting this . . . sort of.

My husband is a great guy and a gentle soul, and he loves me completely, but he can't seem to get comfortable about sex. In the beginning I thought his hesitancy was honorable because he wanted to wait to make it more special. I respected and I waited.

A couple of months into our relationship, we were engaged, and I wanted to test the waters. I made myself look sexy and asked him to join me on the bed. He went down on me and he was pretty good, but it only lasted for a couple of minutes. Then he acted embarrassed.

The times we had sex, I gave my husband head, and he loved it. I have offered many other times, but he says that his brain is cluttered, and he can't have sex unless he can shut his mind down. He can't spontaneously "give in" to my advances, and he is not an initiator. He agrees that he has a mental hang-up. For his benefit, I act like it will be okay.

My husband tells me that he awakes with a hard-on sometimes, and I have asked him to give it to me while I am sleeping, and not to worry about waking me up. But he hasn't and says he's too tired. My husband doesn't want to be pressured, so I leave him alone, and I get hornier.

Recently we had sex one time after planning for it, and it was fantastic! But alas, we are back to the same mode as before.

What a pickle we are in. I would like my husband to know how important it is for us to go to a therapist, and that this is more serious than I let on. How do I get this party started?

An Expert Responds
LAURIE MINTZ, PHD

Jenny, you've taken an important step in acknowledging the seriousness of the problem of a sexless marriage. I agree that the two of you could benefit from therapy. You have tried to resolve this on your own, but it hasn't worked. A good therapist trained in sexual issues could help you work out this issue and grow closer.

Before you talk to your husband though, look at these two beliefs you have: You want to protect the man you love from pressure, and you disregard your own needs by acting like it's okay.

These beliefs are common and understandable. However, shielding your husband by pretending that the "no sex mode" is acceptable is counterproductive. Problems fester when they don't get solved. Not letting our loved ones know what we feel and want may seem easier in the moment, but it damages the relationship in the long run.

Women often put their own needs on the back burner and focus on taking care of others. We tell ourselves that what we want isn't as important as what our partner wants; that we mustn't be "selfish," and the like. Now you need to fully acknowledge and honor your legitimate desire for sex. It's important for you to accept that sex is a vitally important part of marriage, and that you don't need to forsake it because your husband is uncomfortable about facing his issues.

Once you feel centered in this belief, you'll be able to convey your needs clearly to your husband. Talk to him from this position of calm and loving strength. Here are some tips for having this talk.

1. Find a good time to talk, a time when the two of you can focus on the conversation. Maybe tell him in advance that you want to set aside time to have an uninterrupted conversation.

2. Express how much you love him and that a satisfying sexual relationship is critically important to you. Acknowledge how difficult this is to talk about, and that you cannot let this go unaddressed any longer.

3. When explaining how you feel, start your sentences with "I." Say, for example, "I believe sex is an important part of a satisfying marriage," and "I want us to work on our sexual relationship by going to a therapist together." Say nothing that sounds like blaming or accusing. You might jot down a few notes beforehand to stay focused when difficult emotions arise.

Hopefully, your husband will agree to go to a therapist with you. If not, I strongly suggest that you go on your own. A good therapist can give you a safe space to sort this all out and might be able to give you ways to approach your husband that will help him decide to join you in therapy.

GEORGE, AGE 54

My wife, Sarah, and I have not had intercourse for seven years, although she enjoys letting me give her oral sex. The orgasms she receives this way are spectacular, with her entire body in spasms for a long time. It is penetration where we have problems: She says it hurts and, not wanting to hurt her, I always pull away.

Sarah and I had not spent even one night away from the children since our first was born over twenty years ago. I finally convinced her to spend one night at a hotel recently, hoping we could start to turn our sex life around. I packed lube and a sex toy, just in case.

I announced I was going to take a shower, hoping she would do the same. After more coaxing, she did. She emerged. I kissed her and loosened the towel wrapped around her. In this hotel room, glowing from the hot shower, it was the first time she had let me see her naked for ten years. (She'd always put on her nightie before taking off her underwear.)

I pulled her onto the bed and began a long, slow dance of foreplay. I took her over the edge orally, then applied lube liberally. As gently as I could, I entered her, but she immediately winced in pain. Like every other time we got this close over the last seven years, I withdrew.

"There are many other ways you can please me," I told her, and she honestly had no idea what I meant. "You know, with your hands or your mouth." I guided her hand on my erection and started to move it slowly.

"But I don't know what to do!" she said, crying. I stopped.

I felt like I was standing on the other side of a canyon from my wife. I had just seen the elephant that had always been in our bedroom: I realized that whenever we had made love, I had been the initiator. Although our lovemaking had been sensual, with soft kisses and gentle caresses, my wife had always been the receiver of sexual stimulation, never the giver.

"Has it always been this painful for you?" I asked.

"No, but it's always been at least uncomfortable. A few times it's been okay, but sometimes it's quite painful."

We tried again a couple of times over the next few months, with the same results. I wonder how much of the problem is physical and how much is psychological. I know that dyspareunia, painful intercourse, is a very real medical problem. But Sarah refuses to get help.

Now every night we hold each other closely and tenderly before we go to sleep, and we wake each other with another hug and a kiss before we get up. But the elephant is always in the room.

An Expert Responds

MICHELE MARSH, PHD

I'm going to respond to both George and Sarah on this one.

George: You clearly are committed to your marriage and love your wife very much. But you have a marriage that feels celibate for you and does not provide you with sexual satisfaction. Your wife is in touch with her enjoyment of the pleasures of receiving oral sex, and she is upset by her difficulty in opening up to give you the pleasures of intercourse you desire.

I realize your wife has not accepted the idea of getting help, but have you consulted with a relationship-and-sex therapist by yourself to explore possibilities? Many people in your situation would struggle with how to respectfully—and yet assertively—express their needs and frustrations. Engaging in some professional therapy would help you figure out ways to approach your wife with your needs and with your request that she get some help.

Meeting with the best sex and relationship therapist in your area and finding appropriate medical doctors trained in sexology would be a good start. I am sure you would be amenable to attending sessions with Sarah to help her feel supported and to help her find courage to talk about these private

matters. A book to help you look at how you can approach this kind of difficult communication is *Your Perfect Right*, by R. Alberti and M. Emmons.

Although having a more satisfying sexual relationship is clearly important to you, I do not know whether it could become, at some point, a "deal breaker"—that is, so important to you that you would risk your relationship by having an affair. From my point of view as a sex and couples' therapist, I see your situation as ripe with risk—either for increased unhappiness (causing more stress and even depression), or for the broken trust and sense of secrecy that usually follow breaches of fidelity.

You are a patient and kind man, and your generous attitude is a cornerstone of a good marriage. An equally important cornerstone is forthrightness about the importance of your own needs. This can increase the emotional intimacy and enrich the relationship. A sex-and-relationship therapist could help you explore how to discuss with Sarah what you need and "coach" her on how to give you manual and oral stimulation.

Sarah: You and George are a very loving couple who are devoted to your marriage and your children. You are a sensual couple at times, enjoying how George pleasures you with oral sex. I assume you would like to please George too, but the problem is penetration.

Many women experience discomfort during penetrative sex at points during their lives, and there can be many causes for discomfort or pain. The good news is that most causes of pain are subject to definite improvement.

It's important to figure out the reasons for your physical pain. It may seem amazing that sex—a natural function of the body—can be complicated by issues like a variety of medical or physiological events, fatigue, mood, family upbringing, early sexual experiences, and emotional events in marital life. But it is true.

Luckily, there are specialists who are expert at discussing and diagnosing these issues. An expert sexologist can find out if your pain is due to some anatomical or physiological situation and prescribe proper treatments. For certain problems in muscle tone—which can contribute to pain—physical exercises or physical therapy can be helpful. Most of these treatments do not require any medications that are systemic (such as hormone replacement therapies or antibiotics) unless there is an infection requiring a medical cure.

Your own physical health and well-being are involved here. "Use it or lose it" applies to the muscles in the genital area just as to others. You surely deserve to rule out any conditions that may become more complicated going forward, such as infections or pelvic-floor muscle-tone problems.

Many women experience physical changes with aging that complicate their sexual life. These can include changes in vaginal lubrication, thinning of the vaginal tissues, irritation of the urethra and other surrounding tissues, and increased susceptibility to infection. Talking to a professional sex therapist can provide major relief, as you discover that many couples struggle with and succeed in working through these issues within a supportive, professional relationship. This could open new doors in your marriage—and you'll have a happier, sexually fulfilled husband too.

Note from Joan: Please also read Chapter 11 for more on vaginal pain.

BABS, AGE 50
My husband is aging in such a way that sex is not interesting for him anymore—including not being interested in working on improving in that area. But I am just beginning to discover

and enjoy my own sexuality. How can I deal with my feelings of frustration and sadness? I feel that I am being kept from a wonderful jewel of experience in the second half of my life because my partner, whom I still love, is not interested in my sexual exploration. Do I roll over and accept the fact that my sex life is over because my partner isn't willing to get involved?

An Expert Responds
FRANCESCA GENTILLÉ

I celebrate your renewed interest in sexuality and pleasure. When one partner desires more, different, less, or more exploratory sexuality than the other, this can stir up feelings of sadness, anger, numbness, frustration, or even fear, for either one or both partners. I encourage you to continue getting juicy, self-aware, and pleasure-filled. This may ignite something in him—especially if he is not made to feel wrong or pressured.

You might say something like, "I'm beginning to open up to exploring new levels of my sexual pleasure. Would you be willing to help me explore and discover? You can't do anything wrong. It's all good on the path to learning."

If that is not effective, I encourage you to explore additional options, including these:

- Encourage your partner to get his hormone levels tested—especially the adrenals, the thyroid, and testosterone.

- Enjoy on your own your newfound sense of erotic self-mastery. Although you may prefer to deepen and expand your sexuality with your partner, many Tantra and sacred-sexuality books encourage solo exploration.

- Celebrate the other great things your partner brings to your life.

If your needs continue to be different, and he doesn't want to participate with you in your sexual exploration, you might feel pulled toward a relationship outside the two of you. If you're considering this, it's important to have an open conversation with him about your needs. You might ask, "I hear you when you say that you are not interested in sex. I can understand that. I have needs for sexual expression, touch, and physical intimacy. Would you be willing to brainstorm with me about changing our relationship design so that I can explore getting my needs met elsewhere?"

ATHENA, AGE 68

My husband stopped having sex with me three months after my marriage. That was thirty-four years ago. He was great in bed the nine months before we married, but he could never get it up around me after marriage. He said it looked ridiculous when he looked in the mirror while he was making love to me that last time. He stopped in the middle, and we never had sex again. I never said anything to him. It was too embarrassing. We sleep in separate rooms.

I am the daughter of a battered woman. I remember hiding under a table at the age of seven, watching mom being beaten by my brother and dad at different times. She never told anyone or made changes. I was a battered wife in my first marriage. I married the first man I went out with, and he turned out to be a wife-beater. I expected my second husband to treat me better. Instead he was cold and verbally abusive.

I never liked sex with either of my two husbands. It just got numb and painful. I didn't like the smell of his breath or the semen on my body and sheet. It was disgusting.

Now decades have passed without the slightest iota of affection from my husband. I express my sexuality by writing romance novels with tender love scenes. They are published, and all my fantasies are played out in the novels I write. My husband has never read anything I wrote and doesn't want to. I watch midnight TV and movies with sex scenes. I have sex with myself. When I told my husband I had sex with myself, he got angry and chased me out of his room.

I am afraid to have sex with a real person because I don't want to be soiled and don't want anyone poking my insides. I'd be too embarrassed to make it known that I'm still interested in sex but afraid that a partner would cause me pain, as I have an atrophied, prolapsed vagina. Like my hemorrhoids, I just shove it back up.

How do you deal with a verbally abusive husband with a temper when you need his money in your old age to pay the rent, health insurance, and social security benefits? I stay because I have no income of my own. What do I have to look forward to—more temper tantrums when and if my husband begins the long decline into Alzheimer's elder rage?

Is it okay to pleasure myself, or is it toxic to my body at a certain age? Is my health enhanced or not enhanced by sex with myself?

An Expert Responds

ELLEN BARNARD, MSSW

Athena, I thank you for telling your story. I suspect that there are other women who will find it sadly familiar.

I understand that you have not really resolved your past trauma of seeing your mother abused and your own abusive marriage. A good counselor can help you resolve this, even at this point. Seek out free or inexpensive counseling through a service organization that works with victims of domestic violence. Clearly this trauma is still haunting you, and you deserve to move past the intense pain you're still feeling. Once you explore and understand your feelings about what you saw and how your mother handled it, maybe you can put them in a place in your mind that allows you to think of them less often and with less angst.

It is wise to create a fully separate life and self from your husband. There is no reason you cannot create your own life—with friends, interests of your own, and activities that are engaging and rewarding. You do need to understand that you cannot share your feelings or anything about your own life with him. He will just find ways to continue his abusive patterns if you engage with him in any way. Your acceptance of that will help you have a more fulfilling life.

Sexual self-pleasure is very good for both your physical health and your mental health. This is a vital component to taking care of yourself, and I'm glad that you have allowed yourself to do this. Continue enjoying self-pleasuring as often as you wish, and use stories and fantasies.

Will your husband get worse as he ages? No one knows the answer to that, but in general people *do* become more of whatever they already are as they get older. Your husband may become more abusive and difficult, but we cannot predict anything of his behavior at this point.

You do need to prepare to find ways to take care of yourself, even if it means leaving. A domestic-violence specialist can help you find a place to go and the means to support yourself. You deserve to be finishing your life without abuse. If he becomes more difficult, you need to give yourself permission to get help to leave. There is no such thing as "no choice," although some choices seem very difficult and frightening.

It's Over: When It's Time to Leave

Do you stay, or do you go? What if you feel like you're drowning in a life where you feel lonelier *with* your partner than alone? What if all the life and love have gone out of the relationship?

One thing's for sure: If the relationship is physically or emotionally abusive, you need to go. If it's just "not great," try counseling first. If there's still love in the relationship, a counselor can help you find it and work on it. At a certain point, you may say, "I tried everything, and I can't stay."

CHRISTINE, AGE 49

For the last year and a half, my husband of twenty-three years and I have been having problems. It began as his midlife crisis, and he had an affair. We separated for a year, and he saw the error of his ways and decided to come back. The problem is my feelings for him are gone. He says he loves me and wants our lives to be great together. But there is no spark for me.

While we were separated, a wonderful man befriended me and encouraged me to work on my marriage. It was wonderful to talk to someone who understood what I was going through.

When it appeared my husband was not coming back, we took our relationship to the next step.

Then my husband changed his mind. I agreed to try again and said goodbye to my new friend, which was extremely painful. My husband and I tried for three months; however, I realized how much happier I would be with my new relationship. My husband and I cannot communicate well at all. I decided to file for divorce. My husband is very hurt.

My husband and I were never friends to begin with. We slept with each other almost immediately, and the sex was so good that we assumed everything else would fall into place. It hasn't been a terrible marriage, but the ups and downs were constant and difficult. I am tired of problems that never resolve themselves.

I choose to move on, even if my new relationship doesn't last. This was a very difficult decision, but the right one for me. I read many books on marriage, divorce, and relationships, and saw a counselor with and without my husband before making this decision.

I know I will land on my feet. I have grown in the last year and discovered how happy I can be on my own. I feel like I have outgrown my husband. There's no longer any chemistry in my marriage. I would be settling for less than I want, and that is unacceptable.

We make excuses for people's faults while we are falling in love with them. My counselor told me that it takes eighteen months for the adrenaline high of a new relationship to wear off to where things are "normal." Think how many people accept marriage proposals during that time? I did, twenty-three years ago.

MAMIE, AGE 69

The changes in my feelings about sex were related to being with a hostile, negative, narcissistic, angry man who no one in her right mind would want to sleep with. Anger is *not* an aphrodisiac. His potency level resembled that of a garden slug, because that's what anger does to a man. This had nothing to do with testosterone levels.

It is not unusual for women who have been in bad relationships to get into new but equally bad relationships. As Dr. Phil says, "The best indicator of future behavior is past behavior." If all you have known is a lousy relationship, how do you establish a good one?

I knew from the outset that this man was inappropriate for me. He was angry about almost everything that had or had *not* happened in his life; opinionated almost to the point of insanity; neurotic; needy; and critical beyond anyone's ability to stand it.

When you are surrounded by this kind of darkness, it takes over your life. You wake up to a person who is depressed, jealous, and needier than a cranky two-year-old. And you go to sleep with this draining phenomenon as well.

The ironic part is that when you are *yourself* an optimistic person, you feel that you can fix this, that you can make this person happier, that he will snap out of it. Finally, you get it: This has nothing to do with you—except that he is driving you nuts. You didn't cause it, and you can't fix it. You just have to get this person out of your life.

That's what I did. I finally got smart enough to kick his sorry ass out of here.

How to Know It's Time to Let Go

BY TINA B. TESSINA, PHD

I've helped lots of couples solve difficult relationship problems, but it isn't always possible. Here are three reasons to let the relationship go.

1. Your partner keeps going out of bounds. For example, your partner is struggling with compulsive behavior—a sexual compulsion to keep having affairs, spending money on porn, gambling, taking drugs, drinking too much alcohol, or losing money on the stock market. If you've caught your spouse out of bounds before, and he or she keeps repeating the behavior, it's an addiction that's out of control. If your spouse won't get proper treatment, or treatment hasn't worked, leaving may be your only choice. Paradoxically, leaving an addicted spouse is often the only thing that breaks through the denial.

2. Violence or verbal or sexual abuse: If you are subjected to violence, verbal abuse, or sexual abuse, it's important to get safety. Report the abuse, get a restraining order, and get out of the relationship.

3. You tried therapy, but it didn't work. If you and your spouse have been to couples' therapy and have given it a good effort, but it didn't fix the problems, stop your fighting, or teach you to communicate, perhaps one or both of you haven't enough motivation left to stay together.

5

Talking about Sex

"COMMUNICATION IS OVERRATED," posted a member of an online community for women over fifty. "Unspoken communication is the most effective."

I don't think so. I think the combination of spoken and unspoken communication is essential if we are to understand each other.

When we first date someone, don't we do both—incessantly? We talk earnestly, wanting the other to know everything about us, feeling we're finally in a safe place to express our innermost thoughts. We play: We make up games, invent jokes that would be meaningless to anyone else, and share our joy like two kids becoming best pals. And we communicate buckets of emotion through touching, kissing, and holding hands.

Then we get to know each other, and we seem to understand without talking so much. We feel like we can read each other's minds. (Actually, I think it isn't so much mind reading as having already had the conversations that allow us to interpret each other's gestures and expressions.)

Now things may feel different. We're in different bodies, with different needs and wants, comforts and discomforts, pleasures and pains. It's time to re-open the getting-to-know-you phase at this new time of life. We've got to start talking again.

Taking Pillow Talk Out of the Bedroom

When Robert and I fell in love, we talked and talked. We wanted to learn every little thing about each other's opinions, feelings, life experiences, past relationships.

But talking about sex wasn't easy at first. I wanted to show him what I liked; he wanted to discover this on his own. If I asked for something directly, Robert took it as a criticism and felt defensive, and when I was discouraged from asking, I felt shut down. We both wanted the same thing—our own and each other's pleasure—but over the decades of single life before we became a late-in-life couple, each of us had become set in our ways.

We needed new skills to talk about sex. So we learned them. We discovered that if one of us wanted to talk about a need or desire related to our intimacy, the best place to discuss it was *out* of bed—maybe on a walk, or sitting together after dinner with classical music playing in the background. A quiet time, a quiet place, nothing urgent on the agenda.

We also learned that even if the temptation was to argue or defend ourselves, it worked best when we just listened to the other's concerns. Sometimes just "I understand what you're asking for" was enough of a response. Other times we would decide how to work out whatever it was. The process, learning to keep our words gentle and positive, became precious to us.

Four Guiding Principles for Talking about Your Relationship

BY LAURIE MINTZ, PHD

Faulty beliefs about communication can erode relationships, while healthy attitudes can enhance them. These principles for healthier, more effective communication will benefit your sex life and your relationship in general.

- Ask for what you want. Don't expect your partner to intuit what feels good to you. If you want your breasts caressed, let your partner know. If you want your penis stroked, tell your partner.

- Check out your assumptions about what your partner likes or dislikes sexually, rather than operating on beliefs that you have never actually communicated. If you think your partner doesn't like to perform oral sex but have never discussed this, ask directly.

- Work out issues as they arise. If your partner turns you down for sex several times, then talk about your feelings rather than silently holding on to your hurt and resentment.

- Work to resolve issues rather than to win a fight. Rather than to trying to convince your partner to do what you want, discuss your sexual issues, and all other issues, with the goal of better communication, understanding, and enjoyment for both of you.

I Wish My Partner Understood . . .

Some of the saddest comments I get from readers describe sexual issues that are being hidden from partners. This seems so self-defeating. If your partner doesn't know you're unhappy, or needing to be touched a different way, or needing to be touched period, how can anything change?

ADVICE FROM AN EXPERT

Communications Strategies When Your Partner Won't Talk about Sex

BY YVONNE K. FULBRIGHT, PHD, MSED

Humans can't read minds, so you have to communicate your desires in order to get what you want in a relationship. Unless you make your wishes known, your partner is not going to change or even attempt to fill your needs. Here are some suggestions for bridging the communications gap.

- Let your partner know how you feel using "I statements," such as "I miss having sex with you. I am hurt and confused that you haven't wanted to make love." You cannot be faulted for how you feel, and expressing yourself this way is likely to get a more positive reaction than something like "What's wrong with you? You never want to have sex."

- Ask questions that invite discussion instead of yes/ no questions. For example, say "I was hoping we could talk about why we're not having sex anymore," instead of "Are you not interested in sex because I no

➤

longer attract you?" Don't make assumptions, which close off discussion and can cause your partner to clam up.

- Pick a time and place when you can focus on just the two of you. Don't have the conversation when you're doing another task. Plan a downtime when you can create a private space to talk. The more natural you can make the conversation, the less threatening it will be.

- Communicate that you want to work on your problems as a team effort. Do not accuse or blame your partner for the problem.

- Pay attention to your own and your partner's body language. A great deal of what you're saying isn't coming from your mouth, but from your stance: how you're holding your arms, how you're sitting or standing, and your facial expressions. Do you appear defensive? Uncomfortable? Does your partner? Attention to body language will help you to gauge how the conversation is going.

- Ask for suggestions on how to make things better, rather than telling your partner how it should be done. People are much more likely to act on what *they* see as being possible versus what someone dictates to them, especially in an intimate relationship. Let your suggestions come across as just that—suggestions.

KATE, AGE 58

I am still shy about telling my husband what feels good to me. For instance, I rarely climax without manual stimulation, but I have always treated this as my "dirty little secret." When we have sex, I usually don't climax. I still enjoy the act, but if I feel the need for release, I masturbate in private. As I've aged, it's almost impossible to climax without clitoral stimulation—but my husband doesn't have a clue.

I know he'd be more than willing to "help," so why can't I reveal my problem to him? Possibly because I've gained twenty pounds since we met, and I'm ashamed of my body these days. The less he has to touch my chubby belly area, the better. Also, my urinary incontinence pads make me feel ugly and self-conscious. Even when my husband does occasionally feel "frisky," I'm unable to relax and let him touch me, because I'm afraid the pad will turn him off before we get going.

I know we still need to try to express our love sexually, because it was such a wonderful part of our relationship in the beginning. I am sorry I haven't been trying harder to express my feelings and fears. My partner doesn't understand my needs and limitations because I'm too embarrassed to share them with him. So I guess I sabotage our sex life before even giving it a chance.

An Expert Responds

ELLEN BARNARD, MSSW

Kate, your story is more common than you imagine, so I'm glad you had the courage to tell it. It's time to stop having secrets from your husband. By withholding the truth, you are not trusting that he will love and cherish you just as you are.

We often do not share our needs with our partner, fearing that we'll be judged or rejected. If that is the dynamic of your relationship, then you need to address that dynamic, not continue to hide your own needs to avoid your fears. Most likely you will learn that he is delighted to learn about and provide what you desire.

Take the plunge and tell him, "I want to share something with you. I have learned that I need a lot of direct clitoral stimulation in order to have an orgasm during sex. I want to teach you how to touch me so that I can come with you when we make love."

Then show him, or tell him, or bring your vibrator to bed with you (if that's what you like), and show him how to use it, or ask him to make love with you in positions that allow you to touch yourself during sex with him. He'll love seeing your pleasure, and he'll be flattered that you have shared this information with him.

As for your weight, does he look the same as when the two of you first met? If not, do you still love him and want to be close to him? I hear from men constantly that they love their wives, round bellies and all, and that what is most important is to be close, share pleasure, and maintain the intimate bond that deepens the connection.

Have you addressed your incontinence with a pelvic-floor therapist? Many women are able to develop their pelvic-floor strength enough that they no longer need to wear incontinence pads. You are very young to be accepting this, unless you have some anatomical reason that this cannot be addressed through physical therapy.

Regardless, there are ways to make sure that you and your husband enjoy intimate contact. Plan sex dates so that you can void and change into something that makes you feel sexy before initiating sexual contact. Take control of your intimacy so that you are comfortable, and stop avoiding it. For the health of your relationship, you both deserve to have a rich, loving, intimate life together.

JEN, AGE 54

I find myself without passion for my husband of twenty-eight years. I love him like a dear friend. There is no physical intimacy. He thinks it is just a health issue, and that I am not interested. He is still kind and doesn't seem to care that we have lost each other as lovers.

I feel guilty because he's such a kind, dear man, and I have no idea what happened outside of not feeling needed or admired. His philosophy is that no one can make you happy or sad, so there is no praise, admiration, or encouragement. I want a marriage where there is joy in what the other does. He doesn't seem to be interested in sharing his intimate life. I thought that, as our life went on together, that would grow, but it hasn't.

My husband has health issues, and lately it's more difficult for him to keep an erection. He's showed me ways to "make it work" to be satisfying for him: a progression of touching that is pleasing to him. I'm glad he was comfortable in talking to me about it. But sex became more difficult in "trying to do it right." It's no longer a relaxing, fun, close time, but more of a having to think about getting it right—for both of us.

I'm embarrassed to do it wrong and don't want to hurt his feelings if he doesn't get it quite right for me. I don't want to discuss how his "difficulties" make it less fun for me. So I avoid sex, even though I know I miss out on the intimacy that is precious to me and our relationship. He's very open and loving, so I don't know why it's so hard for me to talk about it. I don't want to bring it up, because I don't want him to feel bad.

I'd like him to notice and appreciate me, and not just when we have sex. I'd like to be affectionate and playful all day in small ways, not just "those" times. Maybe he's not sure what I'm thinking and he doesn't want to put himself out there, not knowing if I don't want to be bothered.

I believe sex is so important as we age and it needs attention. Flags need to wave! Long-term relationships need to keep the joy of intimacy alive and in many cases it needs to be found again. My husband and I need to be less Jack and Jill going up a hill and more like those kissing porcelain dolls.

Experts Respond

LIBBY BENNETT, PSYD, AND GINGER HOLCZER, PSYD

Many people share this loss of romance in a long-term relationship and are unsure how to rekindle it and negotiate the changes that come with aging. Your sadness is understandable as you consider your fading desire and the waning of passion in your marriage.

For both you and your husband, hormonal changes are contributing to your loss of desire and to his need for added stimulation. We all face this as we travel that road of life. But you can find ways to reconnect and enhance the passion that you once felt.

First, consider your communication style. Some ways to express yourself will make it easier for you to communicate and will make your words more palatable for your partner to hear. Try to talk when emotions are calm. Avoid serious conversations in the heat of the moment. When your emotions are elevated and the issue becomes tense, defenses go up, and it's hard to get your point across.

We all think and process information differently, so it's important to listen effectively. Try to paraphrase what your partner says to be sure you understand clearly. Ask for clarification so that the meaning of what you are saying and hearing is understood.

If the issue gets too heated, take a break, and agree on a certain time to return to it. Show compassion to your partner. Avoid a diatribe: You may lose your partner's attention if you hold the conversational ball too long. Be careful not to assume that you can read your partner's mind, as that always gets us into trouble. Keep checking out what your partner really means.

Tips for Reconnecting

- Tell your partner you're very interested in a sexual relationship.

- Let your partner know you miss the playfulness of your interaction and would like to rekindle the fun.

- Talk about the types of touch you would specifically enjoy. Show your partner the touch that turns you on.

- Don't make every interaction focused on his erection and orgasm. Include nonsexual touch, massage, playful toys, and lubrication.

- Try using emails, text messages, and the phone to stay connected and sexy with your partner.

- Explore your own body and what feels good at this stage of your life. Keep self-stimulation a priority, and share your discoveries with your partner.

Helping Your Partner Talk about Sex

I often hear from people having sexual problems with their partner. They may want more, less, or a different kind or quality of sex. Although sexual difficulties won't magically go away by talking about them, effective communication is a big first step.

ADVICE FROM AN EXPERT
Good Sex Follows Good Communication
BY TINA B. TESSINA, PHD

Humdrum sex usually indicates a blockage in communication. Hurt feelings and misunderstandings can take away the magic. Once you open up the communication, good sex follows. Here are some secrets to good communication.

- Listen, don't resist. When you don't like what your partner is saying, instead of giving a quick, negative response, listen and think for a few seconds more before responding. Your initial response may change. Even if it doesn't, you'll understand what your partner is telling you. When you later want to express something, you're more likely to be heard when you've been willing to listen.

- Look your mate in the eyes. Make eye contact when you listen. Your companion will feel more understood and cared about, which will change the feeling level of the discussion. Women are much more open to sex when they feel safe. Men have much less performance anxiety when they feel understood.

➤

➤

- Focus on partnership. Remember that above all, you are partners. Check frequently to make sure you're acting like partners, and not competitors or avoiders. You're in this together, and partnership is what it's all about.

Counseling: It Really Helps

I'm firmly convinced that individual counseling and/or couples' counseling would improve the sex lives and emotional lives of 90 percent of the people who write to me. Counselors and therapists know how to help you to cut right to the real issue, to see it clearly yourself, to communicate it to your partner, and to resolve it. Who doesn't want that?

Unfortunately, sometimes one partner won't get counseling. Maybe he or she doesn't think there's a problem, or doesn't want to rock the boat by letting out true feelings and critical information, or thinks a counselor will take the other person's side. I hope this section will give you the tools you need to bring your partner around. Even if your partner doesn't want to go to a couples' counselor, you can go alone.

How to Approach Your Partner about Couples Counseling

BY JEANE TAYLOR, LCSW

Here are a few tips that could help you persuade your partner to seek couples' counseling with you.

- Timing is essential. Plan your serious talk at a time when you're both rested, unrushed, in a good mood, and feeling close. Neither of you should be under the influence of alcohol or drugs, not even a little.

- Tell your mate how much the relationship means to you, that there are problems that need addressing, and that the two of you need some help and guidance, because you've not been making progress on your own. Explain that when one person in a relationship has a problem, the relationship has a problem.

- Explain that you would like for the two of you to get some couples' counseling. Select someone who is licensed in your state to practice psychotherapy.

- If your significant other refuses to see a professional, explain that it is important to you. Find a good couples' counselor and start working on yourself and the relationship on your own. Ask if your mate will go with you twice, for your sake. I've had clients come for couples' therapy even when their partners refused to come. They were successful in making positive changes, and they learned tools to use at home.

RANDY, AGE 59

I still love my wife of thirty-six years, but it's no longer the unconditional love that I used to feel marriage demanded. I realize that I've accepted less, and I regret being so compromising.

We never had sex until we were married, although we had some arousing petting sessions, which mortified my fiancée because she was taught that "nice girls" didn't have those feelings. After we got married, I expected that my kind and understanding nature would make her feel comfortable, and she would become the sexual partner I dreamed about. I ended up being her protector and romantic lover, but even though she feels she has made great strides, her sexual needs are pretty white-bread.

I was pornography and she was a romantic movie. I had to tone myself down, and I wanted her to loosen up. Before we got married, she had never had an orgasm, never masturbated. Now she comes when we use a vibrator, or when I perform oral sex on her. Even though our marriage is solid and we love each other, sex has always been something she has done *to* her, and she only actively participates when I directly ask her to do something. I have always been so thankful that she loves me that I accepted less than what I was giving.

I can no longer just "will" an erection. I need more stimulation and variety. I've aged, and my erections are usable, but not the stiff-to-the-base erections that I need for vigorous thrusting. I realize that oral stimulation of a semihard cock would be wonderful.

I have always desired oral sex. She loves it when I do it to her, but if I ask her for it, she frowns and gags with only the end of my cock in her mouth. That does a number on my now fragile erection, and we both end up upset and depressed.

In therapy, I discovered how naive I was. The therapist asked me directly what I wanted in variety and frequency of sex. I was surprised at what came out, and how freeing it was to finally say it openly, without guilt, to a nonjudgmental person. I grew through therapy, and I don't feel so damned guilty about my sexual desires.

My wife and I started seeing a sex counselor. We have made progress as a couple, and I am amazed that this therapist got my wife to open up and discuss sexual issues. As a result, we are engaging in more intimate contact *not* resulting in sex—which increases the anticipation of actual sex. She has become more open to new things and seems to understand that it's normal for an aging couple to continue to grow and explore, sexually.

We're not over the hump yet. My wife is still not comfortable with most of the play that I suggest, but I'm more comfortable with my desires, and the therapist is getting her to open up somewhat. I couldn't have imagined her ever talking to someone else about sex. It's actually more than I hoped for.

An Expert Responds

KEN HASLAM, MD

As an aging man, Randy needs lots more stimulation—visual, physical, and emotional. Porn, hand jobs, and oral sex from a loving, sexually enthusiastic partner are almost a requirement.

As we age, orgasm is no longer a requirement for having satisfactory sex. Neither is intercourse—penis in vagina ("PIV")—a requirement. Long sessions of total-body touch, genital caressing, kissing, and tender words—combined with the unashamed and practiced use of dildos, vibrators, hands, mouths, and fingers—may well lead to satisfactory sex for both partners, even if PIV (or for that matter, orgasm) never occur.

What must occur, however, is open and honest communication about what is and is not working as a turn-on.

I find that men tend to worry about erectile issues, and women are most concerned with the "heart" connection. Both partners have to ask for what they want. Shared intimacy, shared eroticism, and shared vulnerability are the goals, not orgasm.

Men: With the right partner, limp dicks do not matter, nor does PIV sex. Women: You need to know that caressing a limp dick is very pleasurable to the man, even if it is not "working," and that this does not always have to lead to conventional sex.

LISS, AGE 57

My husband and I have been in a monogamous marriage for thirty-two years. We have enjoyed a vibrant social life, romantic getaways, daily walks and talks, travel, and Tantric workshops. Even with so much going for us, we almost got divorced eight years ago.

A major source of tension was the pressure to have the same level of sexual desire. Since no two brains or hearts are alike, one partner always has a lower or higher level of desire. At times my husband would tell me that I was inadequate if I refused his sexual advances. He needed me to affirm and validate him as sexually desirable. The more my husband kept coming on to me, the less I wanted sex.

Since my husband was often the initiator and I the rejecter, I got to have sex when I wanted it, and on my own terms. He might have been able to pressure me into having more sex, but he couldn't pressure me into wanting him, which was what he yearned for the most. Nobody wants to be the unrequited lover. The more vulnerable he felt, the more angry he'd become with me. In this scenario, I played an equally destructive role. I wasn't motivated to have sex out of desire—I did it when I felt guilty or afraid that he'd leave me.

When the dynamic flipped—when sometimes I wanted sex more than he did—he'd decide that he didn't want it. He didn't dare trust that my behavior would continue. Too many times we'd end up draining each other, getting stuck on opposite sides, defending and arguing about our positions. How could we stop this dance of pain?

During this midlife crisis, we discovered the book, *Passionate Marriage* by David Schnarch, PhD. The approach resonated with us so much that we started seeing a *Passionate Marriage* therapist and attended two of Schnarch's couples' workshops. We were getting a marriage education that our graduate degrees overlooked.

We finally learned how to start by working on ourselves, not each other. Until I could value myself, I couldn't expect my husband to do it. Together and apart, we worked on our anxieties, dependencies, and vulnerabilities. The key was to discover who we are as individuals and what makes us tick— both of which has nothing to do with our partners.

This learning process changed our sexual dance to one of intimacy instead of manipulation. I learned that I must continue to consciously *choose* my partner every day of our lives together; that I must continue to realize the importance of his existence in my life. To increase my sexual desire, all I had to do was face the vulnerability of my choice. Now I find the juice of my sexual desire in the eyes of my husband.

When Should a Couple Seek Counseling?

BY MICHAEL CASTLEMAN, MA

There's no hard-and-fast rule on when a couple should seek counseling. When a problem festers, when you have the same conflict over and over and there seems no way out, no resolution—that's when to consider counseling.

Every sex problem is also a relationship problem, and vice versa. If the main issue is control, decision-making, or conflict resolution, then start with a couples' counselor. If the main problem is sexual—a desire difference, orgasm issues for the woman, erection issues for the man—then I'd start with a sex therapist.

I'm a fan of sex therapy. Studies show that two-thirds of couples who consult sex therapists report significant benefit within six months. That's pretty good. To find a sex therapist, visit the American Association of Sexuality Educators, Counselors, and Therapists (AASECT), www.aasect.org. Click the map of the United States and Canada, and get a list of all the AASECT-certified sex therapists in your state or province. Another helpful site is the Society for Sex Therapy and Research, www.sstarnet.org.

If your partner won't go, you should go by yourself. This is not as good as when the couple goes, but going solo gives you a place to vent. It may equip you with new coping skills that can help you deal with the relationship issues. And you may be referred to some written material (such as my book and others like it), which you can litter around the house in the hope that your partner picks it up and checks it out.

6

Off the Beaten Path:
Nontraditional Sex Practices
and Relationships

NONTRADITIONAL SEX PRACTICES and relationships among the senior set could be a book in itself. Huge numbers of us have broken out of socially sanctioned relationships and made unconventional choices. If you're looking to expand your notion of sex and relationships, this chapter might point you in a new direction. If you're happy with your choices now, I hope you'll still find these glimpses into other people's lives fascinating.

Open Marriage and Polyamory

Many of us could never imagine having an open relationship: Jealousy, we know, would get the best of us. But that's not true for everyone. For many monogamy is just not a satisfying option. And as a couple grows old together, building trust and growing as individuals, they may decide to open their relationship to outside exploration.

The following was excerpted with permission from *Loving More: New Models for Relationships* (www.lovemore.com).

Polyamory is romantic love with more than one person—honestly, ethically, and with the full knowledge and consent of all concerned. Polyamory often involves multiple long-term committed relationships, but it can also come in many different forms.

The point is love, romance, intimacy, and affection with more than one person, openly and ethically, by mutual agreement all around. Polyamory is about sex to the same degree that any romantic relationship is about sex. For some, sex is a driving factor in relationships. For others, romance and emotional or spiritual connection are more important.

Polyamory is not cheating, because it involves honest communication, disclosure, trust, and respect rather than deception. It is not the same as swinging, because polyamory is focused on connection and relationship-building, while swinging is more about recreational sex.

Some people choose polyamory because they are just not wired for monogamy and need more than one love to feel complete as a person. Others simply see monogamy not working very well. Some people feel they find deeper intimacy in polyamory as they explore deep emotions, challenges, and joys.

Many "polys" feel and deal with jealousy. However, polys tend to see jealousy as something to master rather than be mastered by. They are willing to deal with it, talk about it, examine its causes, and see what they can learn from it. Many find that the more they move through jealousies that come up, the easier it gets.

For many, the level of honesty, self-knowledge, and sensitivity to their partners' deepest desires brings more intimacy than they ever experienced in monogamy.

Others may find that involvement with more than one person takes away from the special bond or intimacy they feel being with just one. Polyamory can be a very intimate way of relating and loving, but it's certainly not the right choice for everyone.

DAVID, AGE 70

Faye and I have been married for fifty years. We have had an open marriage with occasional partners for more than forty of those years.

Our first time opening our relationship, Faye and I discussed ideas and fantasies. We invited another couple to our home for dinner and a massage. It was a beautiful evening ending in a passionate sexual exchange. The roof didn't fall in and no lightning bolts befell us. How simple and sweet it was.

We formed an open marriage. Our marriage is the center of a large wheel with long spokes radiating out from the hub. The spokes represent the people who contribute to the hub. Our love for each other expands with each contributing experience. Love multiplies—not divides.

Occasionally, Faye will have a date with someone, a night out. Without jealousy, I get warm when I imagine the progress of their evening. She dates only people we both know and like—no blind dates or bar pickups. Her safety is paramount. The next morning, we discuss the details of her date, and our own intimacy blooms.

I don't own this beautiful woman, and she has chosen to live with me. So it is a pleasure to share her with other nice men whom I know and like. She feels pride in sharing me with women whom she respects. It's also fun to go on a double-date and have a sex-partner exchange, and then later compare notes and share ideas.

All that goes with aging also applies to open relationships. We still see couples we had fun with thirty-five years ago. Some people move away and, sadly, some have died, and we miss and still love them. Sex play slows down with time as our body chemistry changes. We still play, just less often, but with just as much fun.

We both understand that this is adult fun, not a dating game, a home-wrecking endeavor, or affair. It is exciting and rewarding to see how others look at Faye; how they love and appreciate her. Our lives are greatly enhanced by expanding a relationship that is already very good.

ADVICE FROM AN EXPERT

Is Polyamory for You?

BY KEN HASLAM, MD

Entering the world of multipartnering is not easy. But when it works, it can change your life, as it did mine. I am a polyamory activist, and until recently, I had several partners—some married, some not. Of the married ones, their husbands are my good friends. I am now monogamous with a new lady in my life but still have the polyamorous perspective. My sex drive, at seventy-five, is alive and well.

More and more folks over sixty are attracted to polyamory. I have met couples where one or the other does not get their sex needs met by the partner. I see plenty of gray hair in the swing community too. I know one couple where the man is unable to provide enough sexual stimulation for his wife, so they go as a couple to swing events. She gets her needs met

➤

by other men while he watches and sometimes even assists. It works for them, and they have remained married for forty years. Both are in their seventies.

A word of caution. Go slow! Read about it and follow the three commandments of polyamory—communicate, communicate, communicate. Be open and honest with your partner, and ask for what you want. You might get it, and you might not. But not being honest leads to more trouble, not less.

Sometimes the reason for taking a lover is that one partner is no longer interested in sex and the other is. They agree that the libidinous partner should find satisfaction outside the marriage, while keeping the marriage intact.

DANA, AGE 59

I love having orgasms. I have always had a very strong desire for sex, which hasn't changed as I've aged. My husband's libido diminished, and he quit wanting sex or intimacy. We sought medical help, but the Mr. says he is just not interested. In the past I was very strong in my belief about not having sex outside my marriage. But I did not want to leave him, so we jointly decided that I should seek out a lover.

I went on the Internet and found a very caring man. We had a wonderful seven-year relationship. After that ended, I used the Internet again and had many "interviews" with men, but I was not happy with most of them. I did not want a smoker or an alcoholic, and I wanted him to make sure it was not a problem for his wife. I did want a married man, since I was married myself and was not leaving my husband. I am open enough with my husband, who has met my lover. He knows when I go but doesn't want details.

I have so much fun with my current partner. He is caring, thoughtful, and a blast to be with. We try to find time as often as we can. We have an awesome sexual relationship.

JULIANNA, AGE 70

I'm enjoying being loved by two men. One is my soul mate and lover, and one is my husband and longtime friend and companion. Both know about each other. I live part-time with each.

My husband was (and is) a good man, but he was impotent and lacked any sensual inclination whatsoever. After twenty-five years of a sexless marriage, my health began to fail. There are people, like me, who need to be loved—not just a hug, a kiss, or a fondle, but really made love to—to survive. I became sick and depressed. We went to counseling and doctors.

Then I went on a cruise, where I met my soul mate. He had been a widower for five years after a wonderful marriage of fifty-three years. I told him that I was in a celibate marriage. He would have liked us to have become much friendlier on the cruise, but a kiss goodnight was all I was willing to allow at that time. At the end of the cruise, we said our goodbyes.

I came home confused and in a pickle. I was falling in love with my new friend. My biology was going crazy. I didn't think that someone at age sixty-seven could go though the emotional roller coaster of budding love. I could hardly contain myself. Thank goodness I was seeing a counselor and had someone safe to talk to.

I visited my cruise buddy for two weeks, and he became my lover. I have been going back and forth several times a year for the past three years. I'm living a double life—no, an especially full life.

There must be millions of women who are experiencing the same pain I did from a lack of loving. Many of them are in a downward spiral, in body and mind, because of the rules of conduct placed on us by culture, the environment, and ourselves. In the past three years, I've learned more about love and sex than I did in the previous sixty-six years, thanks to the kind, gentle, loving patience of my lover. I realize how lucky I am.

BREENA, AGE 59

My husband and I have been together for thirty years, and my lover and I have been together for two and a half years. The joy we share is emotional and spiritual as well as physical. I'm at peace with my sexuality—I appreciate it, I relish it, and I don't torment myself with questions about whether what I am doing is okay.

When my first husband expressed an interest in having other lovers, I agreed. Once we were in an open relationship, I found I liked it and wanted to continue after my divorce.

I am currently in a community of people who have varying degrees of sexual interaction. I like the freedom of being naked with others, of touching and caressing and playing with sexual energy, without unspoken expectations of what it means or where it will go.

My lover and I became sexual fairly quickly. We went hiking, then he had dinner with my husband and me, and we all talked. Over the next weeks, we developed feelings for each other. He told me, "I'd like to be naked with you." Soon we were exploring each other's bodies. We talked about our feelings and were totally present with each other physically and sexually.

Both my husband and my lover are attentive to my needs and make sure that I'm satisfied sexually. Having other lovers keeps my husband and me from taking each other for granted. We've worked to rewire our brains so that we don't think that jealousy is a sign of love. When we love someone, isn't it natural to want them to be happy and to experience joy?

Swinging and Multipartner Sex

Swinger Sandra Ann enjoys multiple partners and is feeling more sexual than at any time of her life. She sent me photographs of herself posed seductively in high heels and lacy lingerie. She looks self-assured and totally at ease with her sexuality.

SANDRA ANN, AGE 75

In my younger days, my marriages were sexually inhibited. After my divorce at age fifty-eight, I decided it was time to enjoy what my body was made for—pleasure, both giving and receiving. I have been happier ever since. I am multiorgasmic, which I never knew when I was married. It is always exciting to my partner, knowing he can pleasure me so well.

Being single and in the dating game as an older person has been much more exciting and enjoyable than in my younger years. I use numerous dating sites, including some for swingers, and I get many connections. Last year I was in two professional porn videos, and the company wants me back again. Performing in front of others is a real turn-on for me.

At seventy-four, I had my first gangbang. In the swinging lifestyle, a gangbang is a minimum of four men and one female. It is consensual and arranged. It was the most exciting day of my life. I loved the attention all the men showed me. Each wanted to pleasure me better than the guy before. I loved the variety of bodies.

I have since had four more, each better than the last. I set the rules: no anal, no hair pulling, no watersports, no pain.

Light spanking is good; I like that. One was twelve men and myself; it lasted six hours, with the men arriving intermittently.

I have been with men as young as twenty and as old as eighty. Many younger men want the company of a mature woman. My dates all know my age. We exchange pictures, so we both know what to expect.

My biggest problem is bladder infections. My doctor tells me it is similar to "honeymoon syndrome." Since I have numerous partners, the clitoris gets irritated, causing the bladder infections. I am on antibiotics frequently. My doctor does not like the fact that I have multiple partners and says I am addicted to sex. It is difficult to convince him that I am just being me for the first time in my life.

JEZZ, AGE 51

My boyfriend and I are swingers, with the full knowledge and consent of my husband. My husband is fifty-two. My boyfriend is fifty-eight. My husband is disabled, and we have never been able to have penetration sex. We did have oral and masturbation when we first married, but this stopped after several years. For years toys were my only relief. At around age forty, my desire for sex increased dramatically. I started experiencing orgasms for the first time.

Three years ago, I finally admitted that the lack of sex was a huge issue. We agreed that I could find a lover. I started attending swingers' parties, where I met my boyfriend. We started out as sex buddies, but after about six months, we both knew we had fallen in love. This was something my husband had feared would happen. I reassured him that I still loved him and that I would never leave him. My boyfriend has always shown great respect for my husband.

My boyfriend and I continue to attend swingers' parties where we are recognized as a couple. We love our open sexual relationship, and we love the lifestyle. My husband enjoys hearing about the parties—who was there and what happened. For now this works wonderfully for all three of us. What the future holds, I can't say for sure. I am content to take it one day at a time and enjoy what we have.

Elder Booty Calls: Casual Sex and "Friends with Benefits"

When I was single in my thirties, there were men in my life I could call for a friendly, sexy, mutually satisfying romp. We genuinely liked each other but had no expectation of exclusivity or a future together. Sometimes single seniors write me wondering if a sex-buddy relationship is possible at our age.

ARLETTE, AGE 64

I found my regular partner online. I wrote in my profile that I was separated and loved living by myself, that I had no intention to ever live with anyone again, and that the only thing that would add to my good life was regular encounters with a lover. I have had a beautiful sexual relationship with the first one I contacted. I drove at night to his house, fifty-five miles from mine, with an agreement to have sex. Was I crazy? No, just horny, and feeling that I've got nothing to lose at this age.

By far the best thing about sex at this age is how liberated I am. I don't need anyone to "approve" of me anymore, and since sex is the basis for our relationship, we are both letting it all hang out. The complete lack of inhibitions is fabulous. Sex as a younger woman was a way to please a man. Sex now? Well, he'd better please me! Of course, this is a two-way street—I definitely take care of him as well.

I love the orgasms. I use my electric toothbrush, or Persian cucumbers, or big carrots, or my little vibrator. I have explained to my partner that women usually don't come through vaginal sex, and he now watches me masturbate while his head is right there above my clit. He encourages me with whispered sexiness and nips at my inner thighs. The man is beautiful. I think this may last a while.

SETH, AGE 61

I have spent a lifetime discovering who I am, and that I am okay having more than one sexual partner. Something major dies in me when someone wants me to be monogamous. My partner wanted a monogamous relationship, and I completely shut down, sexually. I was not comfortable explaining why.

I don't want to have to choose between two people. I've had a lover for over eleven years where we only get together a few times a year. It doesn't take away from the love but brings more into the relationship.

Sexuality is a powerful energy, and I don't feel one person can satisfy all those needs and wants. It is still difficult to be completely honest with my feelings. I don't feel I have the safety. I would like to learn that I am not the only one struggling with similar issues.

BDSM for Seniors

BDSM (Bondage and Discipline, Sadism and Masochism) includes an array of sexual practices involving power exchange (dominance and submission), restraint, and inflicting or receiving pain. Pain may seem to be the absolute opposite of pleasure to many of us, but for some people, they are intricately entwined, and consensual BDSM play is a thrilling combination for reaching sexual heights.

SCARLET, AGE 66

I identify as leather-queer dyke. I came out into BDSM in 1973 after meeting a powerful woman who was a strong feminist and loved to bottom. Risk and adventure turn me on. I love trying something a little difficult, knowing that working together to pull off an extravagant scene can increase the vulnerability, intimacy, and arousal.

I've been in an open relationship for three years with a woman who is now twenty-seven years old. She is very loving and also very nasty; she has fabulous energy, strength, and daring. We play with piercing rituals, ball dances, energy pulls, canes and whips, bondage, fire, and fantasy scenarios about power and helplessness. We have a closetful of toys. We play with others.

The age difference is less of an issue than one might expect. When we first got together, I was afraid that I would look ridiculous or like a dirty old woman with my young partner, but that didn't happen. My friends have stopped saying, "You go, girl!" as if I had accomplished something amazing by falling in love with a woman fourteen years younger than my daughter.

I usually know people pretty well before we get into bed. BDSM practice is so complicated that it is very rare to have a first date that satisfies all of one's fantasies, so we tend to grow into our connections—and that's what I like, and what keeps me safe.

Early in a date, we talk about what we each need. We don't assume that we already know what the other person likes—or, for that matter, how her clit works. To be a good lover, I have to ask what she needs, and to get good loving, I have to ask for what I need. Occasionally, I need to remind my dates that I am not fragile, so please don't treat me like a teacup.

I love to play for extremely long periods of time, because the change in consciousness becomes more profound. I have some problems with degenerated disks and arthritis, and I get tired earlier than I used to. I can rarely maintain a scene for more than three hours.

I know very few women or men my age who have chosen to live as outrageous a life as I have. I treasure the handful of older partners who gave me guidance when I was younger. Now I guess it's my turn. There is no such thing as "too old" to enjoy sex fully and flamboyantly.

ADVICE FROM AN EXPERT

Safe, Sane, and Consensual: Watchwords for BDSM Play

BY DOSSIE EASTON

"Safe," "sane," and "consensual" distinguish thoughtful, responsible, and ethical BDSM from problematic, harmful, or dangerous connections. These watchwords describe the agreements we need to make in order to safely usher our fantasies into reality.

BDSM fantasies tend to be intense, erotic, and often about danger—we do love scary stuff. To engage in erotic role play, we need to understand the difference between fantasy and reality. We may love the idea of being kidnapped and put in bondage so tight we can't defend ourselves from erotic attack, but to enjoy this luxurious event, we need some way to say, "My left

➤

foot is falling asleep." These occurrences are everyday stuff for SM players, and the response is always to loosen the rope and carry on.

We share clues about what turns us on and what gets us off. Delicious, consensual, erotic dominance and submission require that we get familiar with each other's limits. Whether it's arthritis in my wrist, or a shoulder too sore to swing a whip, limits must be respected.

"Safe"

Physical safety is a must. We must use safer sex to prevent disease transmission. We must learn where it is safe to hit someone with a whip and where it is not (for example, not over the kidneys). Many groups offer classes and workshops to learn how to do fancy stuff safely, from bondage to bullwhips. Both require a lot of practice and expertise—bodies only bend so far, and bullwhips require exquisitely accurate aim.

"Sane"

Sanity has to do with commitments we make to each other when we get intimate, particularly with risky role playing. When we enter into scenes of helplessness or pretend punishments, or when we bring forth our precious inner bully for purposes of fun and fantasy, we are taking emotional risks. We must respect everyone's emotional needs. If either partner gets upset and needs to stop a scene, we absolutely must honor that person's feelings.

SM players place a lot of importance on what we call "aftercare": spending time when the scene is over, perhaps cuddling or just resting, maybe drinking juice or eating snacks.

No encounter is truly finished until we've returned to our everyday state of consciousness, perhaps a little happier.

"Consensual"

BDSM players negotiate consent for the pleasure and well-being of all parties. That requires line-item consent. Negotiation can be an exciting form of foreplay—perhaps going through the toy bag and fondling every item while you tell your partner how you feel about it. This establishes a sexy and positive context for when you need to say, "That toy scares me, no thanks."

Most players establish some form of "safe word" that wouldn't come up in the natural course of your fantasy. "No! No! Stop!" might come up when you actually really don't want your partner to stop, so your safe words have to be more neutral. The words "red," "yellow," and "green" are commonly used and understood. "Red" means "Stop; we need to talk." "Yellow" is a request to adapt or fix something, maybe to make things go slower or lighter, or it could mean "You're way ahead of me—let me catch up." "Green" means go: "I am thrilled! Faster, harder, more!"

Finding Partners

First introductions to BDSM play often occur online. You are basically playing with your own fantasy—which can be erotic and fabulous, and it can teach you a lot about yourself. If you bring a relationship into the real world, complications can arise. You don't know the other person, even if you think you do. Worst case, you could meet someone on the Internet who is deliberately deceiving you.

If you decide to meet an online friend in person, talk on the phone before arranging a meeting. A first meeting in the flesh might be at a coffee house, where you can talk and decide whether to proceed further. I don't recommend bars or dance clubs—the loud music makes conversation almost impossible. Listen to your instincts: If you feel uneasy, don't let your turn-on push you beyond your limits. You can always meet for coffee a few times before hooking up privately. Be ready to let go easily if the person doesn't fit what you are looking for.

People of all ages and sizes are finding wonderful partners on the Internet, at BDSM support groups, or by taking classes in BDSM arts. I am sixty-six years old, and I'm still living a fine, sexy life—wrinkles and all. You can too.

TEELA, AGE 60

Is BDSM appropriate for elderly people? What about us who have just come to this scene? Are we out of our minds? Are we wired differently from vanilla folk?

Here I am at sixty, thinking I have missed out on something. I had the best sex in the late sixties and then got married in 1970. No affairs, no nothing—including sex. My husband was frigid! We divorced, and I married a man eight years younger. Now, after twenty-four years of monogamy, I would like some passionate, rough sex.

I am kicking the traditional traces now. Over the past year, I had phone sex with a Dom [dominant, master]. He is pretty powerful, and the suggestions, control, and commands were new to me. I had a sexual fantasy to be taken by this Dom and to be pushed into the mattress, covered with his body; to be taken and used, over and over. However, he turned out to be a controlling bastard, a very dangerous man. He was "mentoring" me, but he really was an opportunist, a cyberpath, an extreme narcissist. He dumped me, and I've finally kicked his influence.

I expanded to the BDSM scene in the last nine months. I did nothing in the dungeon except watch until last weekend—my first flogging! I cried all through it, but not from pain.

Is "kink" for the elderly?

From Joan: An Update on Teela

One of the joys of writing a book over a period of three years is that I sometimes hear from my interviewees with updates. When I sent Teela my edit of her story, two years after she had submitted it, she responded with this.

1. "I left the BDSM scene . . . without doing anything more than that one flogging."

2. "I rose up on my feet and gave that Dom a good thrashing on my blog."

3. "My husband turned out to be the man I was pining for. One close-up look at that nasty character I let into my life, and I saw what I really had—and still have, after twenty-five years. That is the Great Blessing! One thing I learned: Regardless of your age, you need boundaries, and you shouldn't allow yourself to be pushed around. In *any* lifestyle. Sex can be a predator issue. The most important thing I learned is that self-worth either grows or diminishes. We need to examine closely the influences we surround ourselves with. Age should *never* be an obstacle to this. We should do a lot of self-examination. And that doesn't come

cheap. Sex? It's better than ever—and only with my husband. Now, at sixty-two, I realize that I didn't miss out on anything. I just thought I did. My life is full."

Younger Man, Older Woman

I frequently get some version of this question from my blog readers.

> *"I'm a young man attracted to older women, and I always have been. I find their maturity beautiful. How do I meet and approach older women who might be interested in a relationship with a younger man?"*

Yes, young men are out there, eager to arouse, enjoy, and satisfy older women. Usually their comments are thoughtful and earnest. Occasionally though, I get an email or blog comment such as the following:

> *"hello i am very attracted to older woman (ganny) or mature i want a sex replationchip with one its just that i would love to be in a sexual relationship with no strings attached. unfortunatly i have no idea how to go about this. can anyone offer me any help please"*

No, I didn't make that up. When I hear from young men who are in too much of a hurry to proofread, punctuate, or use the shift key, I wonder what they think they have to offer a slow-burning, older woman? What does their rush to the finish convey about how they would treat us in bed? Rarely (but it unnerves me when it happens), an excited young reader asks me for naked pictures and offers to send some of his best . . . uh . . . attributes. Or someone describes a clearly fabricated encounter with a lust-driven, older woman begging for his gigantic, throbbing member, no foreplay required.

Mostly though, the young men who write me speak reverently of their attraction to older women. And the women who respond to them send me stories full of affection and often love for these young men.

Sometimes it doesn't turn out well (see Carolyn's story, at the end of this section). But then again, sometimes it turns out fantastic.

CAROLINE, AGE 50

We met playing an online role-playing game, World of Warcraft. We never meant to fall in love, but it rolled over us like an unstoppable force. When I found out that I was more than twenty-five years Elliot's senior, I went cold inside. Our conversations in no way indicated the difference of a generation between us! But the bond was undeniable, and all attempts we made to sever it failed. We eventually stopped trying and starting building a healthy relationship like any "normal" couple would.

We resided in two different countries. For nearly three years, we had only video calls connecting us. Intimacy was not a problem through the world of VoIP and webcams. In spite of being unable to touch each other, we spent nearly every day together via the Internet. We talked and dreamed, argued, and cried together. We took turns sharing fantasies as we masturbated simultaneously, afterward enjoying the sweet warmth of the afterglow using our minds and hearts to complete what our bodies could not as yet share. The age difference faded as love took center stage. Our relationship not only survived—it thrived!

After years of waiting, we met physically. Elliot and I wept and fell wordlessly into each other's arms, everything having already been said over the many months of electronic liaison.

I'm in the second half of my life—Elliot is barely halfway through his first. He turns down younger women who approach him, as he truly prefers my more mature and "luscious" curves, as he puts it. He loves me in spite of those moments when I forget what I just said, or when my wrinkles seem more deeply etched in my face than the day before.

We've been a couple for more than five years now, and we're still running strong. Both of us agree that we are in this for the long haul. It's been an adventure and a challenge, and both of us can think of no other person we'd rather stand by to conquer each of these new hurdles.

From Caroline's Lover: Elliot, age 22

Becoming lovers with Caroline simply happened as naturally as you're breathing right now. I never went through a phase when I woke up and said, "Holy Christmas, she's twice as old as I am!" The fact is that Caroline lives with an exuberance and happiness that I am deeply privileged to nurture; something that I'm not sure I would find in any girls my age.

The distance is a challenge, but we've found creative solutions. It took effort to charm her from more than three hundred miles away, but this is like any other relationship, where you can't afford to get lazy after the courtship chemicals subside. A text message from work, a voicemail to let her know I'm thinking of her, or suggestions for our next visit together let her know that I hold her in high priority in life.

Like any relationship, we encounter complications. Her wisdom and experience are sometimes at odds with my wanting to learn through personal experience and to be autonomous.

But with these challenges come the qualities that you don't find in younger women—experience, wisdom, intuition, and a firm grasp of what she wants her life to be.

Our intimacy is severely hampered by the long distance, but we masturbate often over webcam when we're apart, and we have his/hers sex toys to help. Caroline is so in touch with herself and her body that sex between us when we meet is free and loving, with strong measures of raw hunger.

Above all, her pleasure comes first. She needs a great deal of time before her orgasms, which I find an art form. The result is lovemaking that's as honest as it is satisfying for both of us. The challenges that come with having an older woman and being in a long-distance relationship are so worth it. Each problem creates a process that I find utterly invigorating.

AMY, AGE 65

My second marriage was a stormy one. I toughed it out for my daughter's sake, though we fought constantly. We had sex for the last time in 2001, and he never attempted again. Our relationship was so poor that I did not encourage it or care. Sex had barely been satisfactory in the beginning of our marriage, and it was totally unsatisfactory by that time.

The following six years, I was celibate. I never even masturbated. Then—I can't explain what I hoped to accomplish—I put my profile on a dating site. I said that I was married and not looking to divorce, but that I wanted something more. Chris, who was thirty-nine at the time, wrote to me with intelligence, kindness, and intuitiveness.

When we met, I thought my heart would pound right through my chest. He was just beautiful. He is kind, gentle, intelligent, and the best lover I have ever encountered. From the very first night, the chemistry between us has been electric. He is the most considerate lover—he puts me first always. With lovers in my past, it was pretty much quick sex and then snore city. This young man has incredible stamina, and we make love for hours. I have multiple orgasms every time we are together.

After a year of loving Chris, I decided to leave my husband. I moved closer to my young lover and got a new job. That was two years ago. When Chris and I are together, I can barely keep my hands off of him, and when we are apart, my mind is constantly filled with thoughts of him. He breathes life into me and opens me up to new thinking, new tastes, new ideas, new sensations. I am wide-eyed and hungry for more.

Do I have fears? You bet I do. I dread the thought that this can evaporate. But I try to take each day as a gift. I will treasure and appreciate this passion for whatever time I have it. I will live it with all the zest and joy that is within me.

CAROLYN, AGE 53

I'd been celibate so long, it seemed that part of my life was shutting down. I had begun to resign myself to the idea that I might not fall in love again. This made me really sad, because I am very loving and sexual.

My thirty-year-old Caribbean lover became the biggest adventure of my life. We fell in love through emails and Skype calls. We'd been writing and calling for seven months before I traveled to his island to make my fantasies come true. When I arrived at the hotel, I thought, *What the hell have I done? Am I so desperate that I have to travel two thousand miles just to get laid? What if we aren't sexually compatible?* I was also freaked out about the twenty-year age difference.

He showed up, and I knew it was just right. He made love to me like no one had before. He wasn't in a hurry. Being with a younger man who was always hot and turned-on made me feel a lot sexier.

I returned to the United States, and he applied for his visa. I thought I'd never survive the one-month separation, though I had survived for years without sex. Suddenly, I couldn't get enough. He arrived, and we married eighty days later—ninety was the max allowed on his visa.

Things did not turn out as I hoped. Two years later, I'm still supporting him. He now seems self-centered and lazy. He only turns on the charm when he feels me pulling away. Otherwise, he's got the life here in the United States, and I'm paying for it.

These sexy Caribbean romances don't always turn out so great. I'm in a difficult place in my life.

Great Sex . . . But We've Never Met

Thanks to the Internet, webcams, phones, and sex toys, people can have sex of many varieties without being in the same physical place. Given that our major sex organ is our brain, and that we know best how to pleasure ourselves, we can have hot sex with lovers or strangers even while foregoing the real touch of their bodies.

ZARA, AGE 63

I enjoy erotica and masturbation but prefer phone sex with a lover. I have real fears about AIDS, so I've withdrawn from an actual partner at this point. My online friend and I have a private blog on which we share erotica and then enjoy phone sex—no limitations!

I met my phone-sex partner online via a social networking group. I shared my writing and interest in erotica, and he contacted me. I introduced him to phone sex. He is a lonely man, widowed. When I learned he was a former professional singer, I asked for him to sing to me—what a turn-on! From there, a mutually satisfying experience developed.

Just putting two people on the telephone will not result in sexual excitement, especially for older women. I have had two online lovers who totally met my needs. They were aggressive talkers. Many women are not used to talking dirty.

If you have not been a long-time masturbator, you should think long and hard about engaging in phone sex. If you're not familiar with your body and how to give yourself pleasure, it won't happen while talking to somebody on the phone or online. A key issue for older women, in my opinion, is the realization that this is probably not going to lead to any other type of relationship.

Over the phone, there is a tendency to move directly to the sex—no foreplay, no loving overtures from the partner. Phone sex is the reason for the call. If you start talking about daily or relationship issues, then one or the other has to make a complete break and start talking sex.

I was fortunate with my first phone-sex partner. He was wonderfully open, and he had a deep, sexual voice that aroused me. He asked questions and told me what he was doing, and I found it easy to slip into sexual dialogues.

One man told me that I was in love with his voice and really didn't know him. True, I was talking to him in order to be part of a sexual liaison, and this was an easy, safe way to do it. As with any relationship, a woman must learn to recognize if she is in love with love, or with the man who elicits those wonderful loving feelings. Looking back, I'm not sure that I've ever been in love with a man, sad to say.

FRANK, AGE 58

Two years after my last relationship ended, I joined the online world, Second Life (www.secondlife.com), a 3-D virtual world built by its residents. Just about anything you can imagine can be done there.

Second Life offers a bloodless, disease-free way to explore fantasies anonymously, which has a liberating effect. Through a combination of cybersex, suspension of disbelief, and mutual masturbation, I have had sexual encounters with more than 250 female avatars. (I say "female avatars" because the form I was interacting with was female, but I am certain that a small percentage were males at their keyboards.) I've had threesomes, foursomes, orgies, sex with a neko (cat-person: a humanoid with light fur and a tail), elves, and fairies.

Suspension of disbelief—accepting what is happening as real—can lead to a better understanding of self and one's needs and desires, and can be therapeutic as well as satisfying. I am involved primarily with the dominant aspect of BDSM which is, again, a safe and anonymous experience when one need not go to a real-life dungeon.

In real life, I have survived a cardiac arrest and brain damage, a burst appendix, and a bleeding ulcer. I have an acoustic neuroma, which affects both my hearing on one side and my balance in general. I can no longer dance, for instance. So a scenario where I can appear young—where I can dance with my partner and charm her with words spoken or typed, instead of stumbling over chairs and spilling my wine—is pretty ideal. I do miss the touching/tasting aspect of real versus virtual sex, but at this time, this does not distress me.

7

Surviving Divorce, Breakup, Betrayal

D UPED. DUMPED. BLINDSIDED. Some of the stories I've received involve great pain and bewilderment. "How can someone who once loved me deeply treat me so badly?" they ask. "Was I a fool to love this person?" Their minds can't fathom the betrayal.

The stories here are full of regret, and they may pain you to read them. But as we struggle to understand relationships, there's much we can learn.

Grieving a Breakup

The breakup of a committed relationship is a death of sorts. Your loved one is still breathing, laughing, and loving—but not in your direction, and I've heard more than one female survivor of divorce say it would be easier if her mate had died. Being a widow, I'd challenge that—nothing is worse than facing that your beloved will never draw another breath. But I acknowledge that it feels that way, and your grief when your spouse or lover breaks up with you is profound and tortured.

You never know when you'll run into your ex-love around town—arm-in-arm with a new lover—and feel like you've been walloped in the gut with a two-by-four. You avoid places you used to go together—or maybe you go there, hoping, dreading, hating yourself for not shaking free. Maybe you dive into a new relationship and try to lose yourself in sex, or maybe you become a recluse. It's grief, all right.

When she was fifty-five, Erica Manfred's husband walked out on her for a younger woman. After she grieved, she got angry and got even by writing *He's History, You're Not: Surviving Divorce after Forty*. Here she shares her tips for women for getting through the first months of being dumped. (Men: Just switch the gender—her tips are useful for you too.)

ADVICE FROM AN EXPERT

Surviving Being Dumped

BY ERICA MANFRED

The days, weeks, months after your husband leaves, especially if it's for another woman, may be the worst time of your life. Here are some ways to get through it.

Find a good shrink. Whether you're consumed with pain, anger, guilt, or all three, a wise therapist can help you turn a trauma into a turning point. If you can't stop crying or get out of bed or have suicidal thoughts, see a psychiatrist and ask for medication. There's no shame in popping some Zoloft in your time of need.

Don't minimize your grief. In one study of people who were dumped, 40 percent went into clinical depression. But no matter how devastated you are or how long it takes—and recovery time varies widely—you *can* get through this and move on,

➤

as long as you honor your own grieving process. Don't short-circuit it. You don't want to be one of those divorcées who are still carrying on about how her ex ruined her life ten years later.

Let it all hang out. Divorce gives you the opportunity and the right to stop taking care of others and let them take care of you for a change. You can even cry in public.

Depend on your girlfriends. If you don't have supportive girlfriends, go find some—they'll become the most important people in your life. It's okay for a sister or other family member to be a girlfriend. It's not fair to enlist one of your kids, which can be tempting if you're lonely. It's too much of a burden for a child, whether that child is five or thirty-five. You don't want to undermine your children's relationship with their father.

Writing well is the best revenge. Write out the rage. I wrote long, vituperative emails to my ex. One rule: Never hit the Send key after midnight. Write a goodbye letter. It's cathartic to write down every little and big thing about your husband and your marriage that you're saying goodbye to, good things as well as bad. Mail it or not.

Get your body moving. Find a physical activity to combat depression. It has to be something you enjoy, or you're punishing yourself further. Dancing is great. Any outdoor sport that provides speed, like bicycling or skating, is exhilarating. Try kayaking—moving through water is incredibly healing.

Find something that distracts you or makes you laugh. After my husband left, my lifesaver was *Sex and the City*. I discovered the show in its last season and rented the videos of the other seasons. A series lets you get caught up in it for a while.

Become a groupie. Try one of the 12-step programs for group support: Al-Anon if your ex was a drinker, Alcoholics

> Anonymous if you've got a drinking problem, CODA (Codependents Anonymous) if you enabled your mate to mistreat you. Join a grief group for support and perspective from people who have suffered losses greater than yours. Divorce support groups can be pity parties, so watch out for those.

> Get a pet. I'm writing this with my little Jack Russell/Chihuahua mix curled up next to me. Having a warm-blooded creature to cuddle who loves you unconditionally can be enormously comforting, even if he has fur and four legs.

Holding onto Your Heart—and Your Wallet

Being older and wiser keeps us safe in most situations, but we're all capable of losing our perspective and bs-detecting power when love sprays a mist of illusion over our eyes, heart, and brain. Several women wrote me about being duped, conned, and cheated out of their money and their willingness to love again. Most would not permit me to use their stories though, feeling too embarrassed. "I should have known better," they told me.

One was the victim of an Internet courtship scheme that preys on lonely, older women and parts them from their money. It was obvious to her friends and to me that she was being suckered, but she wanted so badly to believe, that she got angry at everyone who tried to protect her. I don't know how the story ended, because she broke off communication with me.

Another fell for the "his millionaire parents were just killed in a plane crash in Italy, and he needs me to wire money so he can bury them and come visit me . . . he'll pay me back after their money is distributed" scheme. It breaks my heart.

If you think you're too savvy to fall for a man who lies and promises you the moon, that's what Jane thought too. I happen to know Jane, and she's a smart, perceptive, well-educated woman. That didn't protect her from the promise of true love and the perfect house.

JANE, AGE 70

I was in a very serious relationship for two years when I was fifty-five. This man—the love of my life—was trim, articulate, and intelligent. We both had master's degrees and shared the same profession. He lovingly pursued me with an open heart—emotionally and physically—with gifts and thoughtful gestures, like flowers, when he came for the weekend. I believed that we were a great match—the best I'd ever known.

We bought a home together. I put down 90 percent of the $40,000 down payment. He lived a couple of hours away. He planned to sell his home and repay his share of the down payment. He would be in my city part-time for three years, and then he would retire and we would live in *our* home together. We became engaged.

As months went on, he kept coming up with excuses for why he had not yet sold his home and repaid his half of our down payment. He became distant, emotionally and physically. I finally confronted him, and he said he wanted out. I had to sell the house, give him his fair share of the profit, and then find another place to live.

Tears are welling as I write this now, thirteen years later. I lost the man who had said that he wanted to marry me, that he cherished me and wanted to spend the rest of his life centered around our being together. My heart was broken. I had two failed marriages before this relationship; I have not dated since. I feel rather broken in the "romantic love department."

I now have a full life of meaningful work, people, and interests, but I am too gun-shy to trust again. I do not have the energy to bounce back if things did not work out. As far as love and sex go, I have bowed out—gracefully, I hope.

Joan Responds

I hope for you, Jane—and for all of you who have experienced heartache—that you will meet someone who is worthy of the gift of your heart. It's hard to keep that heart open after this kind of disillusionment, but it's worth it when the person who really does offer love and is the right match for you comes along. It's never too late for that.

Meanwhile, get to know who you are on your own. Enjoy your own company. Make sure your social life is filled with people who make you feel good when you're with them. Take pleasure in activities that fit your values, interests, and goals. Learn something new. You can be whole and enjoy your live as a growing, laughing, independent being.

Dating after a Divorce or Breakup

Recovery from a breakup takes time. Sometimes we head for the rush of a new relationship too quickly, wanting to heal the pain, to assert how attractive we are, and to wipe out memories. It may feel good for the moment, but there's little chance that a rebound relationship will last or make us happy.

CATHY, AGE 58

I had a baby at age forty-two—the baby died. Then, ten years later, I came out as a lesbian and got into a relationship. My sex drive went into overdrive. She made me crazy with desire. I was with her for six years, and I wanted sex all the time. I had never had such a deep sexual experience, and it translated into the love of my life.

A year ago she left me for someone else. It broke my heart and killed my spirit and my sex drive. Right now my sex life is nonexistent. Will I ever have sex again?

I am going through single life as a lesbian for the first time. Many women did this when they were younger, so I feel at a disadvantage. I am younger-looking and -acting than many women my age, and many of them are just too old for me. Younger women are not interested in dating someone who is almost sixty, so I am stuck.

It's hard to find someone who attracts me. I am very picky and have criteria for someone that I will be intimate with. I haven't found anyone since my breakup. One woman caught my eye, but she was not interested in me. Somehow, the women I like don't like me back. Maybe I don't have a realistic vision of myself, or I am just too old.

Funny thing about Internet dating sites: From the time I see their picture to the time I meet them, the women age ten years and gain twenty pounds. I have had some okay dates—but either I or they felt no chemistry.

I also go to as many events as possible, but if my ex is there, I leave—I can't face seeing her. If she is not, I try to stay for at least an hour and talk to two new people. Sometimes that is hard to do. The lesbian community is not that big, and it winds up being like high school, where everyone knows everyone else.

I am trying to meet women who live within one tank of gas from my city—close enough for weekend visits, but far enough that I won't see them at every event. What would I like a lover to do to turn me on? Show up and want me. I think there are lots of other women out there living quiet lives of silent desperation.

An Expert Responds

GLENDA CORWIN, PHD

Cathy, give yourself more time for healing. You've had bad losses—your partner and your baby—and these have a compounding effect. So take really good care of your physical and mental health. Exercise, talk to supportive friends, see a therapist, join a grief group, and take advantage of any resources to help you work through your losses.

It's good to try "light dating," but don't expect to find the right woman for at least another year. Your judgment could be a little impaired by the intense emotions you're having about your losses. Just focus on broadening your social network.

Instead of clinging to the idea that you're disadvantaged because you came out later, use this as an excuse to ask questions about the "lesbian lifestyle." You'll have some interesting conversations, learn lots of variations, and impress others with your curious mind and good listening skills.

Develop your empathy. We all hate being "lonely and looking." We worry about how others see us, and we want to be accepted. The problem with acute grief is that you can get so absorbed in your own pain that you forget others have needs too. Then you may come across as negative and self-absorbed—not an attractive combination. Put yourself in her shoes, whoever she may be.

Grief takes a long time, and you're not going to feel a lot better anytime soon—but meanwhile, what can you do for others? You'll feel better sooner (and increase your odds of falling in love again) if you're involved in altruistic activities. Women love women who are active and involved in making the world a better place—and you're likely to meet some wonderful women that way too.

"You Cheated, You Lied": Dealing with Betrayal

"What *don't* you tell your partner?" I asked on my blog. This drew Franklin to write to me about his immense feelings of betrayal. "It's only because you've been so giving in your blog that I'm opening up to you about this most intimate issue in my life," he wrote me. And over the course of several emails, he told me his story.

FRANKLIN, AGE 50

I don't tell my partner that I'll never really recover from the corrosive effects of her lying while conducting affairs with three men over three years. It's five years later, and while I've forgiven her, I'll never really recover from her deceit. She doesn't understand that it simply isn't possible for me to really trust her about anything major again. We go on with life, we function, but it can't ever be the same.

She resents it when I feel the need to talk about it, so mostly we don't. We did counseling as a couple about three months after I found out. Counseling was helpful in that it forced her to understand what her infidelity had done to me, and that what I was feeling was normal. But she always felt like the counseling sessions were "beat up on her" sessions, and she resented the probing into our relationship issues and her personal issues that led to her affairs.

Counseling lasted about six months until the money ran out. I had several individual counseling sessions, and that helped me come to terms with my feelings and become functional again.

My wife adopted the attitude "Well, we're over that now, aren't we, honey!" She insists she's "fine now" and "that's in the past." Her defense to me was, "I just didn't think about you when I was out on my dates. It wasn't about you—it was about *me* and what *I* wanted."

The biggest aftermath is my ongoing feeling of betrayal. I don't feel she ever accepted full responsibility for the irreparable damage to our relationship. She seems to think that because she went to some counseling and said she's sorry and feels guilty about it, that all is well now. But the "I just didn't think about you" defense doesn't ring true to me and hurts me deeply.

The fact she had sex with other men isn't nearly as much of an issue now, years later, as is the deliberate deceit. Her affairs were calculated and methodically executed. She would even take my phone calls, interrupting the sex, and lie to me about being out shopping. But she claims that she never thought about how her affairs might affect me if I ever found out. She justified her behavior because I hadn't been paying attention to her and her needs and she needed some emotional relief from a bad time we were going through together—which included financial and health problems.

The intensity has faded. I no longer lie awake at night feeling as if my chest is going to explode. She claims that she's completely happy with her life with me now. But how can a person say she "just didn't think about" the effects on a partner? Did I matter so little?

An Expert Responds

REBEKAH SKOOR, MA, MS, IMFT

Franklin, you've been through a lot of pain and invalidation. I am not simply talking about the three years your wife was engaging with other lovers. The betrayal you feel currently seems to have more to do with her inability or unwillingness to take responsibility for her actions and her lack of responsiveness/empathy to your feelings. Any partnership breached with this intricate deceit would be challenging to rebuild. It sounds like you are trying to do the vast majority of the repair work for the both of you—an approach unlikely to succeed.

When your wife says that she "wasn't thinking about you" while out on her extramarital affairs, I hear that she was not valuing you, or how her deceit was impacting you. Even now, she seems to ignore the validity of your experience. What has she learned? That she can cheat and deceive and end up with a husband who keeps his feelings a secret to protect her?

I suggest you tell your wife that you might never recover from the corrosive effects of her lying. She needs to hear this. Whether or not your marriage continues may depend on whether she can take in this information and start working on rebuilding this relationship with you. If she refuses to do this, you may need to ask yourself whether it's healthy for you to stay emotionally invested in a relationship where your wife refuses to hear, accept, or value your feelings.

If you both make a commitment to do the mutual work of rebuilding, you'll need to explore the following issues with a counselor.

- How in touch are you with your individual needs? With one another's?

- What in your relationship contributed to her sense that her needs were unimportant?

- What was the quality of your communication before her affairs? How did you both contribute to that quality?

- What are the benefits of staying together, based on how things currently are?

- What work would you need to do individually and together to rebuild the trust and value in this relationship?

- How willing are you both to do this work?

I encourage you to look into affordable counseling to help you address these questions. Check into low-fee counseling clinics in your area, and whether your insurance will cover part of your fees. Find a support group to attend.

Valuing your own experience of this betrayal is critical, and finding someone who can help you clarify and communicate your feelings will improve the quality of all your relationships, moving forward.

ADVICE FROM AN EXPERT

After Infidelity: Stay or Go?

BY TINA B. TESSINA, PHD

Affairs are devastating to all concerned, and they demonstrate emotional immaturity. While I don't think you should stay and suffer, I do think a lot of people can wind up happier by staying and doing the work, rather than taking the shortcut and leaving without doing the work. Ask yourself, "Have I done all I can within my marriage to correct the problems and get what I want there?"

Dissatisfaction often grows from resentment, and the root causes can be fixed with the help of counseling. With some work, a marriage can be improved. People often get into "the grass is greener" fantasy and later regret leaving after the damage is

>

done. It's possible that you will find an extraordinary love after divorcing late in life, but most of my clients find the potential partners out there are no better than the ones they left.

Top 5 Reasons to Stay after an Affair

1. Your partner truly recognizes he or she has a problem and is willing to get help to fix it, and to be accountable for rebuilding trust.

2. You two are going to counseling to understand why the affair happened and how to fix the problems.

3. You're getting your shared sex life back on track (if it was off track).

4. You have a long shared history, joint finances, and family ties that make keeping the marriage together worth it (if No. 1 is also true).

5. You still love each other, and it's clearly mutual.

Top 5 Reasons to Leave after an Affair

1. Your partner is in denial, is making excuses, and/or is blaming you.

2. You have had it, and you no longer feel connected. (Be sure this isn't just temporary anger.)

3. You are prepared to be on your own.

4. You either have no children, or they're grown, or you're certain a divorce will be better for them than what's going on.

> 5. Your partner refuses to give up his or her other sex partner.

8

Sex with Myself

"ARE YOU SEXUALLY active?" the nurse practitioner asked me last year, readying me for a breast and pelvic exam.

"I'm sexually active with vibrators," I said, unsure what she was really asking. "I have orgasms, but not partners. Is that what you wanted to know?" No, it wasn't, she explained, laughing. The question was designed to lead to offering an STD test if the answer was yes. We brainstormed possible rewordings of the question.

When Robert was very sick, and for many months after his death, I felt no erotic fire at all. My world was in turmoil. I had lost my great love. I would never touch his face or see his smile or hear his voice again. I felt so profoundly grieved that sexual arousal didn't intrude in my awareness any more than a leaf falling in the neighbor's yard.

Then, as you'll read in the Chapter 16 (the "grief" chapter), my body started asserting itself. My sensations started to surface, and I was amazed that I could still feel arousal. But it was hard to get back to it—most of the time, it seemed like too much trouble to get started. Weeks could go by without the urge.

Finally, I did get started, more for my health than any emotional impetus. And I knew that my ability to enjoy sex in the future would suffer if I didn't get back to nurturing arousal and orgasm. It's up to us to keep our sexuality strong, and that's an important component of health.

Masturbation: The Healthy Choice

When we women were growing up, most of us received no education about how to achieve sexual pleasure. You men were lucky—it came naturally to you. Your penis stood at attention, and it was obvious what to do about it. For women, our pleasure spots weren't so visible or so demanding of attention. We got warnings that sex would get us pregnant, but not much—if anything—about the pleasures. We touched ourselves, or our partners touched us, and, by trial and error, most of us discovered the sparks that ignited desire, pleasure, and orgasm.

So what's the point, at our age, of a chapter about masturbation? Three huge reasons:

1. Our bodies change as we age, often requiring more or different kinds of stimulation to achieve arousal and orgasm. We have to rediscover—sometimes reinvent!— our pleasure triggers all over again. The only foolproof method of keeping up with those changes and not letting sexual pleasure fade is to keep touching ourselves to explore anew what our bodies need and desire.

2. Many of us are without partner sex, either by choice or because of the death or illness of a partner, or due to a divorce or separation. These solo periods may be temporary, or they may last for a very long time. The "use it or lose it" advice applies here to both sexual pleasure and sexual comfort. We have to keep having sex in order to stay sexually healthy, and that may mean sex with ourselves.

3. For men, the ability to engage in penetrative sex may become unreliable or even impossible. (See Chapters 13 and 14 for information about erectile difficulties that we need to understand.) Both men and women can compensate and find ways, alone or with a partner, to enjoy pleasure from touching and oral sex. Women, however, mustn't skip penetration altogether, or our tissues will become thin and fragile, leading to lesions and burning sensations. Using fingers or a dildo will help keep our vaginas healthy. (More about that later in this chapter).

ADVICE FROM AN EXPERT

Reasons to Keep Your Sexual Self Alive and Functioning

BY ELLEN BARNARD, MSSW

First: If you think you may want a lover sometime in the future, it's important to keep the nerves firing off, so that you are able to respond when you want to. This system requires regular activity to stay vital and healthy. Second: Orgasms are good for your mental and physical health. At least one orgasm per week, either alone or with a partner, will help you in several ways.

- You'll be maintaining good pelvic-floor health. Orgasms are a pleasurable way to exercise the muscles that keep your internal organs in place and which prevent urinary and bowel incontinence.

➤

➤

- Your risk of depression will be reduced. People who enjoy one to three orgasms per week reduce their risk of mild-to-moderate depression by 30 percent.

- Your immune system will get a boost. People who enjoy one to three orgasms per week have a reduced incidence of colds and other viruses.

- Your risk of heart disease will be decreased. A study found that the risk of heart disease was reduced by 36 percent with at least one orgasm per week.

Sexy Celibacy

Candida Royalle appeared in twenty-five porn films before her feminism led her to pioneer a whole new type of erotic films. In 1984, she founded Femme Productions, the first company to make adult films that spoke with a woman's voice. Now, at fifty-nine, Candida Royalle is currently unpartnered and keeps her sexuality vibrant by pleasuring herself. She shares her thoughts about self-pleasuring.

ADVICE FROM AN EXPERT
Staying Juicy and Fit During Celibacy
BY CANDIDA ROYALLE

People assume I have a nonstop, fabulous sex life because of my work in erotic films and women's sexual empowerment. Since ending a serious relationship two years ago, though, I have not been sexually active. Call it hormonal changes, different interests, or needing time alone after a breakup—I haven't felt the urge to find a new mate.

What I have been committed to, however, is having a date with myself at least once a week to exercise my PC (pubococcygeus)—muscle, which runs along the pelvic floor and surrounds the entire vagina. Then I reward myself with a nice little session of self-pleasuring.

After menopause, sexual inactivity can cause the vaginal muscles to weaken over time. Exercising that muscle, however, keeps the muscles strong and fit and can help prevent problems such as urinary incontinence or a prolapsed uterus. As for helping to maintain a pleasurable sex life, the act of repeatedly contracting and releasing the PC muscle brings blood flow to the vaginal tissues. This helps us lubricate and prevents thinning of the vaginal walls—two of the main reasons intercourse can become painful with age. Bringing blood flow to the vaginal tissues also helps us feel more sensation, so we experience greater pleasure and stronger orgasms.

It's important to make time for ourselves when we don't have a partner. I have an ongoing date with myself once a week to do my Kegel exercises with my Natural Contours Énergie vaginal barbell. I use a weighted barbell for the same reason

➤

one should add weights to any workout routine: It creates muscle resistance, making the workout more efficient and bringing faster results. The time you need to do your Kegels depends on the condition of your vaginal muscles. Once you have improved your vaginal tone, you can usually get away with a maintenance program of once a week. (It's always good to consult your doctor.)

You can do your workout without self-pleasuring, but there are also many health benefits of pleasure and orgasm. When we have an orgasm, we release a cocktail of beneficial chemicals into our system, including endorphins—our bodies' natural opiate-like substance that makes us feel good and boosts our immune system. So I give myself that little reward at the end of my exercises.

Self-pleasuring puts a smile on my face and makes me feel alive and ready to meet the day. Being without a lover doesn't have to mean going without the joys and benefits of pleasure. If and when that lover does come along, I'll feel confident, knowing I'm juicy and ready to take him on.

CHRISTINE, AGE 49

In my early twenties, I'd still never had an orgasm, so I set about it with a Waterpik. When I finally climaxed—and it took a long time—it was incredible. Ever since, I have made jokes about my Waterpik. I love it! It's cheaper than a sex toy, no parts to clean, no batteries, and I don't have to hide it. Plus it has all those wonderful settings! Sometimes I like it softer, harder, quicker, slower, direct, or indirect. I am almost fifty now, and I still use my Waterpik.

Betty Dodson, "Grandmother of Masturbation"

Maybe Betty Dodson can't claim to have invented masturbation, but she led the movement for women to talk out loud about it, figure out how to do it, and applaud the results. For twenty-five years, she led workshops teaching women how to view and appreciate their genitals, and use sex toys to orgasm. Now in her eighties, Betty writes about sexuality and is still a staunch supporter of masturbation.

ADVICE FROM AN EXPERT
Hands and Toys for Orgasms at Any Age
BY BETTY DODSON, PHD

My second book, *Orgasms for Two*, was written while I was having an affair, in my seventies, with a much younger man. I'm now eighty-one and have dropped partner sex for now. But masturbation, dildo play, and hot, dirty fantasies are still pumping out some very good orgasms.

One of the most important ways to continue being sexual is to masturbate. Partner sex for older people might pose problems, due to physical disability or the lack of an available partner, but making love to ourselves is readily available and highly desirable.

We can also share masturbation with a partner: Each person doing him- or herself, or taking turns doing each other. The erotic hand job breaks us out of our rigid conditioning that says there's one right way to have sex: the man on top with a "boner," holding back until his beloved comes and then finally coming himself. That's not likely to work for either the older

➤

male or female. Her vaginal lining is too thin, and she seldom if ever had an orgasm from the "missionary position" anyway. He can't perform like a stud because he has lower back problems and he needs more direct stimulation to get and keep an erection.

So now they can finally relax, and share a sexual activity that works for both of them. Most likely that will be manual sex, oral sex, or sharing masturbation.

Several male clients in their late sixties and seventies came to see me because they were no longer getting fully erect and wanted to know if I could advise them on new ways to masturbate. This is where sex toys come in handy.

Men can masturbate with an electric massager on a soft penis while consciously working the PC muscle. With one hand on the shaft of the penis, the other hand moves the massager around and over the glans, shaft, and testicles—however you like it—with or without a piece of fabric to soften the vibes. By rocking the pelvis, breathing out loud, squeezing the PC muscle, and having a hot sexual fantasy, sexual feelings and sensations will break through to produce a diffused, different kind of orgasm, with or without ejaculate.

No one has to be stuck living a life without orgasms. Pleasure belongs to anyone who is willing to take responsibility for creating it. Here's to all of us older folks having many happy orgasms.

VICKI, AGE 72

Now at seventy-two and with no partner, I masturbate weekly, sometimes with a handheld showerhead on massage-impulse alone, sometimes adding a dildo; sometimes with a dildo and a vibrator. My clitoris is losing sensitivity, but my vagina is still quite sensitive, and the combination of vaginal and clitoral stimulus works best. It usually takes up to ten minutes to orgasm.

ADVICE FROM AN EXPERT
How Self-Pleasuring Helps Partner Sex
BY CAROL QUEEN, PHD

Women who can't have an orgasm during intercourse should start by paying attention to what does make them come.

You may not be aroused enough, or you may not be getting enough direct clitoral stimulation. The easiest way to remedy this is to give the clit extra stimulation via your own fingers, your partner's hand, or a toy—either a clitoral vibrator or a cock ring with a clitoral stimulator built in. But starting intercourse before she's aroused enough makes it difficult for a woman to come, and may be uninspiring, nonorgasmic, or even downright painful and unpleasant. Take plenty of time with what our culture calls "foreplay."

Many women and their partners do not know what will work. I always recommend that a woman learn about her own body on her own, through self-exploration and self-stimulation.

When you stimulate yourself, you learn which types of touch feel the best and how long it takes to feel really good—without being distracted by a partner's presence. As nice a distraction as it is to have a lover in bed with you, many women

➤

> do not focus on themselves and their pleasure very well when there's someone else with them. Masturbation lets you take your time and learn your body and your responses. Then you can share what you learn with a partner.

Sometimes the amount of stimulation it takes to get aroused enough for an orgasm is greater than the amount we get during partner sex, or even alone, using our hands. Using a vibrator may make the difference between "almost came" and "definitely came!" Vibrators offer strong and consistent stimulation. Many people think a vibrator is supposed to be used vaginally, to stimulate the way intercourse does. But optimally, most women prefer clitoral vibration, or a vibrator on (or near) the clit and a vibe or dildo used vaginally or anally at the same time. Using two toys like this has the advantage of accustoming you to penetration while being erotically stimulated and coming to orgasm.

EVELYNN, AGE 65

To me, self-pleasuring is a must! It is my sensual meditation, and I do it often, no matter who or how often I choose to invite another into my lovemaking. Being my own best lover brings me into a place where I know I can offer an invited partner a Wholeness of Self that comes from embracing and loving *me*.

Men Speak about Masturbation

I said earlier that masturbation seems so simple for men compared to women. Even as I wrote those words, I wondered whether it's as easy for men of our age as it used to be. Being the brazen sexuality writer that I am, I emailed this question to a couple of male friends who had always been open to talking about sex.

As men age, do your masturbation habits and techniques change, reflecting new needs and preferences? This is something I don't know and need for my book. Clue me in, would you?

I submitted the same question to my *Naked at Our Age* Facebook page (which I hope you'll "like") and got a rush of responses—some with thanks for bringing this and other senior sex topics out in the open. The following are a few of the responses to my question.

TINGGI, AGE 61

I usually masturbate in the morning. Guys often get a morning erection—a shame to let it go to waste. If I'm not dead tired at night, I will masturbate then also—it's good training for evening opportunities for sharing. I have moved away from the rapid pump jerk-off. Now I lie on my back, fantasizing intercourse, using gentle and prolonged stroking, like what I'd receive vaginally. I usually use a condom to eroticize condom use. Up until my early fifties, I could go from zero to orgasm in about five minutes. Now it takes about twenty minutes.

Facebook Post Reply #1

For me the question is not if change happens, it is how. Men are generally depleted by orgasm (classical "big" ejaculation orgasms). In general I prefer not to ejaculate because of the energetic pit I fall into afterward. I have come to adore the inner power of accumulated chi/kundalini/juju that results from avoiding big orgasms and appreciating the smaller, multiple orgasms. Extended sensuality beats a depleting quickie virtually every time.

Facebook Post Reply #2

I masturbate maybe twice a month, but a hard erection is more difficult than before, due to my prostate cancer treatment. My orgasms are dry, since there is no functioning prostate gland. The effects of the cancer are the only change in my habits and technique of self-pleasure. I would like men and women to know that there can be sex—both solo and together—after prostate cancer.

9

Unlearning Our Upbringing: Women's Stories

A s a girl, I was taught everything about how babies are made and nothing about why we *choose* to have sex—nothing about attraction, desire, satisfaction, or lust (except male lust, which was taught as something to avoid triggering).

And—I laugh because it's so ludicrous—I was taught nothing about female orgasm, or even that the clitoris exists. Neither our local library nor my father's medical library had any clues as to why women might enjoy sex (other than as a means to becoming a mother) or what organ held the answer to the mystery.

I wonder if the reason the word "clitoris" has two accepted pronunciations (CLIT-or-is and cli-TOR-is) is that several generations of men, women, teachers, and doctors never said the word aloud.

My father was an obstetrician and saw many teenaged girls' lives derailed by pregnancy in the years before abortion was legal. It was drummed into my sexually vacant mind that boys wanted to have sex and that girls had to stop them, because it was the girl who suffered the consequences. I had no idea—until a shockingly wonderful, three-hour kissing session with my first love in the tenth grade—that girls *could* feel aroused. That was never part of my sex education. I never had an orgasm until I was nineteen, although I started having sex with my boyfriend at seventeen.

Many of the people who shared their stories for this chapter were stuck in their upbringings for many decades. Most have found their way, educated themselves, and shaken off horrible memories, negative self-images, and bad relationships that happened for the wrong reasons. Some are bitter about the lack of information and misinformation they received in their youth. It's enlightening to read their stories now and to see how their ideas about sexuality have matured.

Overcoming Ignorance, Repression, and Guilt

Women of our era grew up knowing little about sex, feeling shame about our sexual feelings, and—unfortunately—sometimes subjected to abuse or violence. Often our sexuality in adulthood was formed by these negative influences. But if we're willing to do the work and make changes, with aging comes wisdom, which allows us to move on and forge a future of our own choosing.

KATE, AGE 58

I grew up with a tyrannical, abusive father who scared me to death. He made me a shy, nervous girl who was depressed and insecure. My mother, who feared and hated my father, told me that sex was highly overrated and that men use it to control women. She hated sex, and this colored my perception.

When I reached puberty, I had an enormous sex drive, but always felt ashamed of this. I lost my virginity at fourteen and had twenty sexual partners by age twenty-two. I never once enjoyed sex during this time; it was all about getting a man to love me. I needed a man, any man, to provide the love I was lacking. To get a man to love me, I needed to have sex with him.

My father sexually abused me once when I was sixteen. I blocked it out of my mind for many years. Then, one day in my early thirties, I read a story about a woman who was abused by her father, and it all came flooding back.

At twenty-two, I fell madly in love with a man who taught me to enjoy sex, but still I felt guilty, because we weren't married. We broke up after four years. I married a man on the rebound, for all the wrong reasons. I never truly loved this man and hated having sex with him. This produced more guilt, because I knew I was ruining our marriage. After twenty years of living like roommates, we divorced.

Two years later, I had a nervous breakdown and finally got the medications and counseling I needed. My newfound self-esteem led me to meet my current husband. I have been head-over-heels in love with him since our first meeting, and sex with him has been wonderful. I think we both were love- and sex-starved! The best part for me is the complete lack of guilt when we make love.

We are both middle-aged and have wrinkles, saggy skin, and graying hair—but it doesn't matter! We truly love each other—what better way to share our love? Now, in my fifties, for the first time in my life, I enjoy sex without guilt.

TORY, AGE 65

I was drawn away from sex by my religious teachings and drawn toward it by my own body, so I was abysmally ignorant. I got pregnant at eighteen. I was so ignorant that I thought one had to *want* to be pregnant in order to *get* pregnant!

I had an illegal abortion without anesthetic. The doctor was under threat of losing his license if anyone found out that he was performing abortions. The pain almost knocked me unconscious. The agony of not crying out through such pain—so that the other patients in the waiting room would not be alarmed—was one of the hardest things I have ever done. The bleeding afterward almost sent me into shock.

The father hightailed it out of town as soon as he heard, with an "I hope you're okay." After that, the threat of pregnancy made me extra careful, and I think I shrank away from men as a consequence. I was attracted but afraid.

I left the church and delved into travel, education, and a profession. I didn't bother to form an attitude about sex. I just did it, though I still felt it was wrong. The risk of pregnancy continued to be a major threat to me. I was assiduous in the use of my diaphragm.

Then I read *The Happy Hooker*, by Xaviera Hollander, and my attitude changed. Sex was good. Sex was fun. Nobody was harmed by a little nookie. Even extracurricular sex was not such a bad thing. It was much more fun if it was tailored to your taste, and nothing should be out of bounds, as long as nobody was hurt.

Now I teach in the Unitarian/Universalist OWL (Our Whole Lives) program, in which children are taught the facts of life at different ages. The little kids are taught the basics, with sex becoming more detailed and serious as the kids get older. They learn about birth control, the way the body functions, homosexuality, legal considerations about sex, dating, relationships, what makes a good marriage, and how you get there. The kids are treated with respect, and they have fun, as with the Condom Olympics, during which condoms are blown up and never burst, illustrating how safe they are.

As a teacher in the OWL program, I teach what I wish I had learned as a child. I would have had much more respect for myself as a sexual being. I doubt I would have had my unintended pregnancy and abortion.

SADIE, AGE 71

The only sex education I received as a female was in high school PE, and the teacher sexually molested me. She was the first one I stood up to and said, "Keep your goddamn hands off of me." She was not my first predator—there were several in my childhood, including my brother. Standing up to this teacher was the beginning of knowing I had to learn how to take care of myself on my own.

I had sex for the first time at fourteen, with a woman who was eighteen. It remains one of the most exciting memories of my life. She was gentle and kind. However, as I grew up and moved out into a homophobic world, I began to take on fear and self-loathing about being lesbian. I joined the Navy in 1957, when I could be dismissed and shamed publicly for being a lesbian. My sexuality felt like a mixture of wonderful feelings that were often shut down by shame.

I succumbed to society's homophobia and shut down sexually. I tried to pass as a heterosexual in the service, terrified of being found out. I became depressed, anxious, and afraid.

After leaving the service, I had three long-term relationships. I was totally closeted in the first one, came out within the feminist movement in the second, and finally came out publicly during the last one.

It wasn't until 1996 that I decided to be alone and on my own. I got to know myself and really did come out sexually, striking down the demons of shame. Therapy helped me sort out who I was and how I got so confused and hurt about being sexual. My therapist helped me understand my anger and rage. I began to own my right to be myself, no apologies.

I've been asked if being sexually molested by a woman made me a lesbian. Being sexually molested doesn't make you anything but scared and confused. All of us are who we are because we were born that way—a part of the mystery and gift of life.

My path to sexual pleasure and freedom came through understanding that I had to give myself permission to own my desires, fantasies, and sexual feelings. Now I love who I am as a woman, and I can experience the joy of finally setting myself free, at age seventy-one, to fully enjoy sexual pleasure. I have a dream of a healthy, fulfilling relationship with another woman, full of fun, laughter, and joy. She's out there. We just haven't met yet.

NELL, AGE 53

Sex was beyond the edge of the map where "there be dragons" as far as my parents were concerned. They never spoke of it. I grew up suspecting it was a bit wicked. I wish I'd had some early sex education from sources other than high school boys, or the girls I met at pajama parties. My mom gave me a booklet from Kotex when I started my period, but I really had no sex education whatsoever until I sought out Planned Parenthood in college. I would love to have had a book like *Our Bodies, Ourselves*, which I discovered in college, earlier on. It took many years, unhealthy relationships, and therapies of various sorts to unhook those old tapes and free me up to play and enjoy sex.

JULIANNA, AGE 70

I grew up innocent and naive. My parents never mentioned anything about sex, and all my friends were as ignorant as I was. I was a virgin bride when I married at age twenty to a man who was an extension of his penis. He got most of his jollies from the ladies who got paid, and from our live-in babysitter. If he had been a gentle teacher, it might have been different.

Instead, he got it wherever and whenever he could. One day, he said that he was leaving to go visit his sister. That was a lie. I was thirty-six, with no college education, no work experience, and four children.

SCARLET, AGE 66

I was a teenager in the fifties and had to struggle my way out of a lot of repression and fearfulness. In my first years of sexual activity, I thrashed around a lot, trying to figure out things that should have been made known to me, like what a clitoris is designed for, and why it should not be ignored.

ALFIE, AGE 56

My parents were very strict. My father was of the opinion that boys wanted "only one thing," and my mother did not want her teenage daughter in unchaperoned situations. My father threatened to disown me if I ever lived with someone outside of marriage. I never saw much affection from my parents—to each other, or to me—so I had no understanding of healthy adult relationships or sex. When I finally did have relationships, I let people walk all over me. If I had the power to change my upbringing, I would change the strictness, which still makes me inhibited when meeting or being with men.

Surviving Rape

It's bad enough when our early sexual experiences are joyless. It's far more devastating when our first experience is rape. Women often spend their whole lives trying to learn to empower themselves to enjoy their sexuality and to trust men again after a violent attack.

MELISSA, AGE 63

I lost my virginity when I was nineteen by date rape. Immature and young, I was drinking at a party. A guy who I knew was sitting outside the bathroom when I came out. I put my head on his shoulder and said, "I am so drunk." He took me into a bedroom, took off my panties, and entered me. When he was done, he left the room quickly, and I threw up all over the floor.

The next day, I saw him, and he completely ignored me. I felt like a bad girl, dirty and at fault. These emotions festered for a long time. I didn't say anything to my parents, as I was afraid that I would be blamed. Back then I would have been. Date rape hadn't been named yet.

My parents were prudish and controlling and refused to discuss anything that had to do with sex or body parts. They handed me a book called *Growing Up* that discussed mostly animals and fish. I thought that sperm swam across the bed while the couple faced each other and somehow made it into the mother. There was only one short paragraph that dealt with humans, and I quote, ". . . only humans do it in a more loving way."

I became part of the sexual revolution. That was about screwing as many people as you could. Many girls with my upbringing didn't think twice about jumping into bed with someone. Rebellion was the name of the game. We were striking back at society in every way we could, and what better symbol than to have lots of sex with people we barely knew. I thought that rebellious sex was a lot of fun, but I never had an orgasm back then. Most guys didn't know how to pleasure a female. Toward the end of that era, it got to be oppressive that every guy assumed he could get laid.

Sex has changed for me since then. I married for the second time in my thirties, and my husband and I have been together for thirty-three years. He has been so patient with me sexually. After two bouts of lung cancer, eleven years apart, I have learned how much he truly loves me, and that has opened me up even more to him.

My first experience with sex, through date rape, really hurt my ability to trust men. My husband showed me how to trust again. I've come to know what feels good and what works for me. Now, sex is making love with my husband, and it is about a trust and a love that I didn't know existed.

CYNTHIA, AGE 57

I wish my father hadn't tickled me, from the time I was two, to the point where I would black out from screaming. I'd tried asking him to stop, and asking my mother to get him to stop. When I was twelve and stronger, I kicked him hard enough to whiplash his neck. He spent two weeks in a neck-traction pulley and never tickled me again. He switched to elbowing my breasts, which were just starting to grow and were very tender. If I'm accidentally tickled in sex play, I'm turned off for the night, and if anyone ever did it on purpose, they'd never see me again. If anyone reading this has a coparent who tickles a child excessively, get yourself and the child away from the creature!

When I was twenty, some guys raped me, cut me up, and discussed the possibility of murdering me. Friends who had been raped told me they lost interest in sex for months afterward. So I decided to go out and find a brother to have sex with the next night, in keeping with the principle that if you fall off a horse, you get right back on. I was determined to let the good feelings drive those bad feelings out of that part of my body before they could become lodged there.

I went to a park where a lot of hippies hung out and found a hippie who had gotten strung out on heroin and was just at the beginning of trying to get off it. It was the perfect combination: I needed someone who would go slowly, and that's the only way someone with heroin in his brain can perform. One thing he needed for his prospective new life free from smack was to know he could still please a woman sexually, and I was very pleased. It worked great. I never had to go through that long period of not wanting or not enjoying sex.

At some point in my recovery, I realized that in traditional societies all over the world, someone entering adulthood has to endure an ordeal that is terrifying, agonizing, and life-threatening. If they survive it, they prove they can pull their own weight, and they are given adult status. If they show courage during the ordeal, they start out in adulthood already having honor. While the men were raping me, I'd decided I couldn't just lie there and take it. I made fun of them and succeeded in embarrassing them, even though I was afraid that what I was doing might lead them to get mad and decide to kill me. So I was a fully initiated into adulthood with honor.

BABS, AGE 50

My father always told me, "You play with the bull, you get the horns." He lectured me that if a woman gets a man sexually excited, there is no stopping him—and it is always the woman's fault. I still struggle with this programming.

I was cornered and molested at age twelve by one of my father's friends. When the incident came to light, my father chose to keep the friendship with the man intact, and the issue was ignored. I was still required to accompany the family on visits to see this man. I was terrified that he would touch me again, although he never did. What made me sick was the fact that everyone acted as if nothing had happened. There were friendly hellos, smiles, and jokes. I felt abandoned and without any defenders, alone and naked in a dark, hostile land.

I spent the next decade feeling as if the wolves were just around the corner, ready to tear me to pieces. Every time a young man smiled and wanted to put his arm around me, I felt panic and literally ran. I left the high school prom without warning when I saw several boys put their arms lovingly around their dates and pull them closer, hoping for a kiss. Due to my previous family programming, and knowing that there was no one to defend me, normal sexual exploration at that age was squelched by terror.

JEZZ, AGE 51

I was a victim of sexual abuse from age eight to fourteen by two close family members, my father and my paternal grandfather. Neither was aware of the other's abuse. This affected my ability to enjoy sex as an adult in a huge way. I married my first boyfriend at age eighteen, and by age twenty-six, I had four sons. I was married for twenty years to my husband, but our sex life was spasmodic and unfulfilling. I never experienced an orgasm the whole time we were married.

No Guilt, No Guidance

EveLynn's experience was unusual for our age group: She was raised without restrictions. That doesn't mean her coming of age was easy, but many of us may envy how little she had to unlearn.

EVELYNN, AGE 65

My upbringing gave me no values to overcome, and no taboos were placed upon me. But by the same token, I was not given positive guidance either—just no guidance. My appetite for sexual experiences often made me think I was abnormal—I loved sex with my husband, and my friends were always trying to figure out how to get out of having sex with theirs. Through the right opportunities and doors opening, I came to understand that sexuality is an amazing gift—it's one's life force. Now, life turns me on. Hot hunky men turn me on. Courageous people turn me on. Working with soul-mate energy turns me on. Heck fire, I am always turned on!

10

Unlearning Our Upbringing: Men's Stories

EVEN AT FIFTY, sixty, or seventy, men are trying to overcome their upbringings. They are confronting the "I am my penis" idea, which doesn't serve them anymore—but it's more than that. Men who are willing to learn and evolve are coming face-to-face with the need to let go of the machismo they spent so long learning, and to discover a new way to see themselves and male sexuality.

Becoming a Man

It isn't just women who are damaged by their upbringings. Boys of our era grew up with an idea of "how to be a man" that was just as destructive. When men write to me about their experiences and concerns, they often preface their current concerns with their background, to help explain how early influences relate to what they're coping with now. Jed Diamond, PhD, is a psychotherapist specializing in later-life issues, especially for men. Jed was willing to contribute his personal story, as well as his professional tips for letting go of old beliefs about sex and relationships that serve us poorly at this stage of our lives.

JED, AGE 66

I moved into my sexually active years in the late 1950s and early 1960s. Boys learned that girls weren't much interested in sex. Since we boys were very interested, it was our job to break down the girls' resistance and get them to go along with our desires. It was the boy's job to try and "score." It was the girl's job to keep pulling our hands away, keeping her "virtue" intact. Pleasure and joy never seemed to be part of the package.

If you were very lucky to find a girl you could coax, you did everything you could to get to "first base." If successful, you tried to "steal second." After that, you weren't sure what you were supposed to do. But you knew it was incumbent on you to try and make it all the way.

Most of my young sexuality wasn't spent with girls at all, but with airbrushed images from magazines and imagined scenes from forbidden books like *Peyton Place*. In my fantasies, these dream lovers would do all the things that real girls, I believed, didn't want to do. Masturbation became a consistent means for expressing my young sexuality.

Meeting my wife and finally having sex after we had decided to get married, I entered a new phase of sexuality. I found that women not only enjoyed sex but would take an active role in initiating and sharing it. It was a time of sexual exploration with a real person—both of us willing.

As I've gotten older, sex has changed. Sometime in my midforties—the time I've called "male menopause"—sex became awkward and confused. We became like shy, pimply-faced teenagers again. We seemed to have totally forgotten the ease of sexual intimacy and pleasure. We couldn't seem to kiss without our noses getting in the way. Sex was hit and miss. Erections would disappear at the most inopportune times. They would jump to attention when least expected.

This was the most stressful period of our marriage. I alternated between wanting my wife with all my heart and feeling that I should leave the marriage and find someone more compatible. She seemed to feel the same way.

As we moved into our late fifties and sixties, sexuality settled into a new phase. For the first time in my life, I wasn't driven by the need for intercourse. Our sexuality became more playful and less focused on orgasms.

Sex changed—from being synonymous with intercourse, to being any act that creates pleasurable orgasms, to being anything that is mutually pleasurable and creates more intimacy between us. Sex started to include holding hands while we were sitting on the couch watching television. It included unexpected looks of love and longing that would bring tears to my eyes.

Though sometimes I'm nostalgic for the old days, it's actually kind of wonderful to be a man in his sixties with a woman in her sixties, still trying to figure out what it's all about.

That was Jed, the man looking back on his boyhood. Now Jed Diamond dons his psychotherapist hat to pinpoint old beliefs that men have to let go of, in order to mature and relate to their partners on a different level.

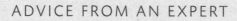

Letting Go of Old Beliefs

BY JED DIAMOND, PHD

Old beliefs can keep us stuck, unhappy, and unable to grow. It took me some time to let go of these:

- "If I'm not trying to have intercourse all the time, any-time, day or night, there must be something wrong with me as a man."

- "If I'm not the aggressor all the time, she'll think I'm not attracted to her."

- "If I accept sex as more loving, touching, and feeling and less 'wham bang,' it will mean I'm losing my man-hood and becoming 'feminized.'"

- "If my men's group found out how little we were 'doing it,' I would lose face."

- "If I can't get an erection on demand, or if it takes longer to get one, or if I lose it before we can have intercourse, I'm a failure as a lover, and she'll probably look for someone else."

- "If her body doesn't look like the models I remember when growing up, I should look for someone who is younger, prettier, and easier to impress."

- "If I go for days or weeks and don't think about sex, I must be getting old and decrepit, and the next stop is Alzheimer's and the nursing home."

➤

> I've come to appreciate that sex is an important part of life, but it is not the be-all and end-all. It's more important to feel a loving connection with my wife and with my life. Rather than being restricted to sexual intercourse, sex has expanded to include all the ways we can enjoy the dance of intimacy and pleasure.

RANDY, AGE 59

Although I had a safe and easy childhood with a lot of adult attention, I learned a warped, old-fashioned view of life, sex, and marriage. The message I got from the church and my mother was that sex—though we never said the word—was for procreation only. What message does it send to people when the most important woman in the church was a virgin, and Mary Magdalene was viewed as a repentant sinner?

Damn, how they messed with our minds—although to them, it was for our own good. Throughout my childhood, my mother taught me how bad I would make them feel if I got in trouble. I never wanted to be a delinquent, but I wish I could have felt the freedom to take a few more chances.

The greatest shame imaginable was unwed pregnancy. The message was never sympathy for the people whose lives it changed, but how ashamed their parents must be. In high school, when a girl got pregnant, she just disappeared. We all knew why, but nothing was ever said. How sad.

When I was eleven and my mother was pregnant for the last time, I got a short talk from my father concerning some vague way that a father put a seed in the mother and a baby resulted. I could feel how uncomfortable my father was, and that was the extent of my formal parental sex education. The remaining education was from my friends and the street.

When I learned to masturbate, I was amazed at how good it felt to touch myself and become erect and use my hand to bring myself off. The fact that boys can actually watch themselves come and connect the rush of orgasm with the spurting of their semen is something that girls miss out on. It's no wonder that throughout their lives, men like to watch themselves spurt.

Masturbating became a furtive activity followed by shame, because in my religion, anything sexual was base and shameful. I was so confused. How could something be bad if it gave me such incredibly wonderful feelings? This environment set the stage for a lifetime full of mental sexual conflict.

As humans, we have the ability to make each other feel wonderful by doing something that doesn't cost anything, is not taxed, is not politically controlled, improves our health and sense of well-being, doesn't pollute the world, and provides us with such intense pleasure that nothing else compares to it. Yet we have managed to twist it around to include guilt, control, and shame.

REDHAWK, AGE 62

A sex-positive education should be mandatory in grade school as well as high school. I would have appreciated been told by adults that masturbation was ordinary and to be enjoyed; that self-pleasure was desirable, good, and healthy; that men can create their own definition of what it means to be "masculine" and can be true to themselves in expressing it and discovering what it means to be a sexual human being.

First Sex

David is a loving partner in a long-term, open marriage—you already read some of his story in Chapter 6. Here he shares his first partner sex experience:

DAVID, AGE 70

From the age of fourteen, I lived the two-faced life of a young male. I was the clean-cut, shy, and proper kid—the kind mothers trust their daughters with. We did no more than kiss or hold hands on dates. But the vision and the drive to run the whole course got hotter and stronger. Finally at age nineteen, I started dating a girl with the same fantasies. We agreed—we would go "all the way."

The big opportunity arrived. It was a perfect, warm, sweet-scented, spring evening. We had been out on a late date. I drove quietly down her long driveway, lights and motor off. The house was dark, and she led me to an unoccupied rental unit.

She unbuttoned her blouse, took off her bra and her shoes, and lay back on the couch. I slid her skirt up to her armpits. I took off my pants as she whispered, "Hurry up." My penis was harder than it had ever been. She guided me into her vagina, but as her pubic hair tickled my erection, I came on her tummy, her pubic mound, and her mother's couch.

At that same time, her mother's voice sounded at the top of the stairs, just out of sight, "Honey, it's time to call it a night."

Unlearning Male Myths of Sexuality: In Robert's Words

Robert was a dancer and an artist by the age of two. Even before puberty, he was taunted by his classmates, who branded him a sissy because he was graceful and contemplative and went to dance class. Is it any wonder that when he was trying to under-stand his own sexuality, he was confused by the male role he was supposed to take on? He told me that he practiced walking like other boys—tempering his dancer's gracefulness to adopt the swagger of a cocky adolescent—in order to fit in and be teased less.

Robert believed completely in this book you're reading now, and this chapter was special to him. Sometimes he would say, "Hey, you need to talk about this in your book," and hand me a yellow legal pad filled with pages of his handwritten notes. I feel honored that the rest of this chapter is in Robert's words.

A Boy Learns about Sex

What's the big deal? I thought. *You have this thing hanging down from your body that gets hard when you play with it* (and secretly I played with it often), *you stick it in somebody, you thrust your pelvis back and forth, and that's all there is to it.* I thought of it as a tool—not a whole lot different from the drills we were using in wood shop to make our birdhouses. I knew about sex and felt quite smug about my clued-in status.

I learned quickly there's a lot more to having sex than build-ing a birdhouse. I learned from a friend that this thing hanging down needed to be handled responsibly, or I might get myself in trouble—that the shy girl everyone pretended to ignore was starting to "show," and my friend was the culprit. Sadly, he and the shy girl were no longer in school.

I now had an idea where my life could take me if I misbe-haved. Not to misbehave meant not to have sex. But it didn't take long to learn that other guys were being credited with a lot more life experience than I was. I felt out of the loop.

The "tool" analogy resurfaced. Only this time, it was a tool of conquest, something heavy-hitting, like a hammer or even a pistol. Bang, bang. Hot damn, thank you, ma'am. Chalk up another one for the stud on the team who was hung a lot better than I was. *It must be terrific to be so well endowed,* I thought, observing this guy slowly strutting from the shower to his locker, hiding nothing, while I kept a towel handy and acted as if I had to dry off quickly in order to get to my job at the bookstore.

Fortunately, using a condom (a "rubber" in those days) was part of being clued-in. Just owning rubbers was a sign of having made it to the big time, and you knew who had one at any given moment. Condoms were bragging booty, a sign you were "doin' it."

I figured out that if I asked one of the key suppliers with sufficient urgency in my voice, the word would get around that I was "doin' it" too. It cost me a dollar. I carefully opened and examined this prized object. Then I hid it in my sock drawer and kept it there for months, even though I knew if I kept it in my wallet and flashed it now and then, I would have scored a few points with one of the uninitiated.

Pretty soon, this game I was playing became boring. There was not a macho bone in my body, although I had learned the "male" way to run, walk, throw a ball, and grab my crotch when it might impress. I wore uncomfortably tight jeans and uncomfortably tight jockey underwear. Occasionally, like the others, I wore a jockstrap under my jeans, since this was the thing to do to avoid embarrassment if aroused. The language we "real guys" shared went something like this: "Shit, I got such a hard-on when Betty Sue got up to give her report that I'm really glad I wore a jockstrap, or everybody would have known."

I liked girls. I liked them as friends, especially the smart ones. I hung out with them, didn't feel any pressure to have sex, made myself available as a dance partner for the ones who would never be asked by the "real guys," had a great time, and got labeled a sissy. I know now that the female company I was keeping allowed me to be myself, particularly my emotional self.

With one friend, there came the time to "do it." Although frightened, we did it together, an act of exploration and discovery. We weren't lovers; we were friends on the way to adulthood. I felt relieved to have the pressure off and at the same time to have a secret so fine, so humanly real. The beautiful young lady who lovingly took me close in friendship remains only a faint memory today, but she opened a door to my knowing that I would never have to prove I was a man by overwhelming or baiting a woman.

I thought it was my penis that would unlock the maleness I have enjoyed for decades. In reality, the key was my willingness to be a sissy.

A Man Learns about Sex

There was still much I didn't know. I could have used some coaching. A woman, I thought, would enjoy sex if I enjoyed it. My pleasure would show how attractive I found her, how I wanted her. The fact that I didn't feel the need for conquest did not erase the self-centered feelings that seemed my entitlement for having a penis. Orgasms, preferably more than one, would leave no doubt to my partner that she gave me pleasure, and that should give her satisfaction. This ego-centered attitude was left over from "the jockstrap days."

Coaching came late—after one loving wife, two children, and one divorce. It came from a woman who showed me what she liked, and put my hand there. At first my penis felt underutilized. Clearly it was no longer top dog. Skin became the essential organ. Oily massages, swimming naked, making sexy underclothes from silk scarves, and learning belly-dance moves kept the penis on call, in anticipation rather than expectation. Foreplay took on a new definition. I felt I was going to sex school.

Other sex-knowledgeable women came into my life. These teachers led me to deeper, more real sexual satisfaction. I was not always a grateful student. I sometimes felt talked down to or treated like a hired hand. While my learning was not always comfortable, that period is full of insight for me now.

My teacher was the woman who moved my hand from her breasts—which I saw as the prize part of her body—to her clitoris, saying, "I'd rather have you do this."

My teacher is my wife, who tells me, "I love your body. You're the handsomest man in my world." When I protest that my stomach isn't as flat as when we were dating, she says, "You look so good to me just the way you are." If you've never heard that, you've missed something. I hope you say it to your lover— it's important.

At our age, we have to separate the useless myths from the reality of what aging is handing us. As long-lived persons, we have enough material to create, inform, and manifest a new story.

What I Know to Be True Now

At our age, we need to be searching for the authentic experience. "What I believed is no longer true for me," we can begin to say, as we gain life experience and grow. "This, instead, is what I know to be true." The aging process forces us to say, "I've got to find the real way. The myth is now so far beyond my grasp that it is futile and ridiculous to attempt to reach it." We might call that the wisdom of sexuality.

In my late fifties, I began to feel I had burned out on sex. Not because I'd had it so frequently, but because I'd been so intense about finding the best way to express my sexuality authentically. I needed a drastically different direction to my life. I began to give my work as an artist undivided attention, and I longed for a time of deep introspection. I went into the woods to live and work. It felt wonderful to be alone, as if engaging in a monastic exercise.

After emerging from my nearly three-year retreat in the wilderness, I met the woman who is now my wife. At age seventy, I am having very good sex, and I continue to learn what pleases a woman. I respect the importance she is giving our mutual sexual pleasure.

We both have health problems that sometimes get in the way, not the least of which is my confrontation with cancer and chemotherapy. I am blessed with a strong body and no sexual-functioning problems. Most of all, I am blessed with a long life that has been enriched through sexual expression and good partners.

A year after writing these words, Robert died of multiple myeloma. It is both joyful and distressing to reread his words now—joyful to remember his beautiful dancer's body, his vibrant sexuality, his commitment to authenticity; distressing to reflect on how cancer robbed him of his physicality months before it took his life. By continuing to showcase his art at www.robertriceart .com and preserving here what he wrote for us, his legacy lives.

11

When Sex Hurts: Vulvar/Vaginal Pain

I GET UPSET WHEN I read Internet message boards where a woman complains of so much pain during intercourse that she avoids sex altogether, and other women rally to help by telling her about this cream or that. Yes, we need lubricant, but if pain persists even with a good lube, there's something more going on, and you need to find out what and why before you decide how to treat it.

If you're a woman who experiences genital pain—inside or outside the vagina, all the time or just during penetration—one chapter in a self-help sex guide will likely not be enough to resolve this. I hope that, with the expert advice I've gathered here, you can get some information, strategies that may ease the pain, and resources (at the end of this chapter) for seeking medical help.

A special thanks to Ellen Barnard, coowner of A Woman's Touch—a wonderful sexuality resource center based in Madison, Wisconsin—for her generous, expert help throughout this chapter.

Get Thee to a Doctor . . . and Perhaps a Therapist Too
This chapter offers some strategies that can remedy many kinds of discomfort. Realize, though, that many kinds of vulvar and

vaginal pain are *medical issues* with a cause that requires *medical intervention*. So first consult a doctor to get a diagnosis. It might be one of these conditions:

- High-tone pelvic-floor dysfunction: the pelvic-floor muscles that support the vagina, bladder, and rectum become spastic and tense, and cannot relax.

- Vulvodynia: burning pain, generalized or localized to the vulva and vagina.

- Provoked vestibulodynia: burning pain at the vaginal entrance when it is touched.

- Interstitial cystitis: inflammation of the bladder's lining, which causes urinary urgency, frequency, and pain.

- Dyspareunia: any pain associated with intercourse.

- Bacterial vaginosis: a form of vaginal infection characterized by a thin odorous discharge due to an out-of-balance shift in the vaginal ecosystem.

Some disorders affect the skin of the vulva and vagina; others make penetration painful because they either affect the muscles surrounding the vagina (the pelvic floor) or they affect the bladder, resulting in pain during deep penetration. Other conditions that don't seem genital-related can affect your sexual experience, such as type 2 diabetes, which can lead to repeated yeast infections.

Since the effective treatment differs depending on the cause, it's essential to get a correct diagnosis. That's often difficult, because many healthcare providers are unfamiliar with sexual pain and are slow to identify the cause or to give a diagnosis. This can be frustrating, but it is important to educate yourself, to be your own health advocate, and, if your pain is not resolved, insist on a referral to a specialist.

Vulvovaginal-pain specialist Susan Kellogg Spadt, PhD, CRNP, is Director of Sexual Medicine at the Pelvic and Sexual Health Institute of Philadelphia (www.pelvicandsexualhealth institute.org). I attended a presentation of hers on vulvovaginal pain at the American Association of Sex Educators, Counselors, and Therapists (AASECT) (www.aasect.org) conference in 2010. Her take-home messages about sexual pain were the following:

- Pain is usually real—it's not "in your head."

- Although not usually life-threatening, the pain is quality-of-life threatening.

- History-taking and accurate diagnosis are key.

- The majority of cases can be managed.

MARLA, AGE 66

My sex life with my boyfriend now is nil. We've been together four years. Sex was fine at first, but then I developed a pain in the vaginal area, as well as quite severe itchiness. Now I cannot tolerate vaginal penetration, and we have pretty much stopped trying or talking about it.

My doctor initially prescribed a steroid cream that seems to have made it worse. A second doctor, a year or so later, said I shouldn't have been using it as often as I was. No solution so far. I'm on oral hormone-replacement therapy, and I am now trying a vaginal estrogen insert. I tried the "e-ring" but didn't like it, nor did it seem to make a difference.

The itchiness is all the time, not just during sex. Sometimes I think it's getting better, but then it comes back. The pain is only when I touch a certain area—an area critical to intercourse.

I know he's frustrated that we don't have sex, but we haven't really had a heart-to-heart talk. He's not too keen to listen or discuss the issue. We don't seem to communicate all that well with regard to this problem, and since my libido is practically nonexistent at this point, I haven't pushed it. I say things, almost in passing, about my "issues," but he doesn't respond. Silent type.

It's just as much me not saying anything as him. Again, the low libido makes me not care all that much. Then I think, *Well, if he cares so much, he should bring up the subject himself and ask me questions*. I've known him almost all my life, and we get along extremely well, even without the sex. But sex is the elephant in the room. I keep thinking I'll get the talk started, but then it's just easier to carry on without saying too much. I know I need to pursue the doctors more. I get tired of going to appointments, and with the low libido, it's not high on my list.

An Expert Responds

ELLEN BARNARD, MSSW

Marla, you need to find a good vulvar-pain specialist to figure out what's going on with your skin. Itching can be a lot of different things, and I'd encourage you to get it addressed, regardless of libido, as you feel it all the time, and I suspect it's affecting you more than you realize. Pain and itch may be related or may be separate. It really depends on what's going on. I know you're tired of dealing with it, and I have great sympathy for you in that regard. It takes many women a long time to find a healthcare provider who can figure out these complex vulvar pain and itch issues.

As for you and your boyfriend, the question is how to start the conversation. It sounds like he is not going to bring it up. Maybe he's perfectly content to have your companionship. Maybe he's happy not to have to think about whether or not he can get erections. Or maybe he's just afraid he'll hurt you.

Of course, he may just be one of those men who are uncomfortable talking about topics like intimacy and sex.

Regardless, intimate contact is important in relationships. It's part of the glue that keeps you close and in tune with each other. The hormones that get released during all kinds of intimate play keep the two of you connected. So you both deserve to have a conversation that allows you to get this out in the open, and to come up with solutions that accommodate your discomfort but still give you ways to be intimate.

Rather than being passive and waiting until he's so unhappy that he feels compelled to talk about it, I encourage you to bring it up in a very neutral way that acknowledges that you know it's an issue, and that you want to talk about it so that you can, as partners, figure out ways to work around the pain and discomfort. Tell him that you're struggling to talk about this difficult topic, but that you think he and the relationship are worth it. Find ways to lead the conversation to a positive outcome that affirms your affection for each other and helps you discover ways to be close that meet each of your unique needs. A good counselor can help facilitate the conversation.

An Update on Marla

I sent Ellen Barnard's response to Marla so that she wouldn't have to wait until the book comes out for this helpful advice. Marla just wrote me that they have resolved their relationship problem, had "a nice date on Sunday and ended the drought," and has been getting medical attention. "So there is a good ending here," Marla writes.

I love it when that happens!

How Can a Therapist Help with Vulvar/Vaginal Pain?

BY LORI ANAFARTA, MA, LAMFT

Vulvar and vaginal pain can wreak havoc on your sex life and set the stage for relationship conflict, avoidance of sexual contact, negativity in sexual attitudes, and the lowering of your self-esteem and mood.

You need to seek out professionals who are knowledgeable in the area of sexual pain. An integrative approach is the best way to maximize your treatment's effectiveness: a gynecologist who specializes in vulvar and pelvic pain, a physical therapist who specializes in pelvic-floor therapy, and a sex therapist or relationship counselor who specializes in women's sexual health. A therapist who works with women having sexual pain will be an invaluable resource in helping you find the right medical professionals.

Painful intercourse has an impact on your whole relationship, and couples commonly come to therapy because their sex life is in shambles. What is happening in your relationship—and how the two of you are handling your emotions and interactions—can have a significant impact on your pain experience. Your partner may unintentionally contribute to the problem by interpreting your pain to be an indicator of lack of interest in having sex, lack of attraction, or lack of commitment to your relationship. Most women believe that they are the problem and expect individual counseling, but ideally, both partners benefit from attending therapy. Both are affected by the woman's pain and the relational issues.

➤

Communicating with your partner about sex can be difficult. You may be afraid to hurt each other's feelings, so you struggle with the best way to say things, or you avoid talking about it altogether. This communication barrier can lead to emotional and sexual disconnection and enduring unpleasant sexual experiences. A therapist can help you learn to talk about sex in nonhurtful ways.

Couples struggling with painful intercourse commonly stop relating to each other sexually. Learning to reestablish a sexual connection can help diffuse anxiety. A sexual connection doesn't have to be intercourse. Holding hands, kissing, hugging, or flirting with each other can help you feel more connected to your partner. Deemphasizing intercourse can reduce the pressure you may feel to perform sexually.

In therapy, you'll learn more about relationship conflict resolution, anxiety and stress reduction, regulation of emotions, and coping practices. The goal is to help you both feel more comfortable and satisfied in your relationship as you work through the medical issues.

A sex therapist can be the starting point for helping you to find, contact, and coordinate the consults with the gynecologist and the pelvic-floor therapist. As you are consulting with those professionals, the therapist can explore with you how your sexual expectancies and moods impact the pain experience. This combination will help you to understand how you work, both emotionally and physically.

MIRIAM, AGE 57

My husband had a serious accident that affected his libido. We didn't have sex for the last five years of his life. I wasn't feeling very sensual myself, because I was in survival mode, keeping our family together.

When my husband died, I mourned him deeply for a year and couldn't imagine being in another relationship. Then I came out from the fog, took up dancing, and fell in love with another dancer. I was surprised and delighted.

But the most horrible thing happened—intercourse was unbearably painful! How and when did that happen? I never had any problem before. Newly in love, my sexual desire and arousal came roaring back, as did my natural lubrication. Why was it so painful? Since I entered menopause during the last years, I wasn't sexually active with my husband, and I had no idea of the changes going on in my genital tissues.

After all those years of no sex, I was deflated to have this problem at the beginning of a new relationship. My lover showed immense kindness, patience, and confidence that it would all work out. While we waited for my tissues to get pliable again, we had a great time with luscious, extended foreplay and making love in nonpenetration ways. Looking back, it was a great intimacy-builder for us.

I worked with a wonderful women's health specialist/physician's assistant, who said that my vaginal tissues had gotten fragile and atrophied. She told me it really was true that you "use it or lose it," and that in essence, I had "revirginated," in terms of being too tight for a penis to make it in comfortably. She introduced me to the Estring, which solved the problem after about three to four weeks.

This specialist was great, because 1) she immediately recognized the problem for what it was (my early-forties female general practitioner didn't have a clue), 2) she said millions of women have this same problem, assuring me I wasn't a freak, and 3) she knew how to fix it. What could be better?

She also helped me immeasurably because she was the first one, after forty years, who used the right-sized speculum for a pelvic exam. Hello? You mean they could have used a smaller, pain-free size all this time? I was both relieved and furious when I found out.

Taking Charge of Your Vaginal Health

After a year and a half of celibacy following Robert's death, I was relying on clitoral vibrators and slim insertable vibrators to keep my genitals healthy . . . or so I thought. When trying to insert a slightly larger sex toy (1.5 inches in diameter, no wider than an average penis), I discovered that I couldn't do it. I couldn't get it past my tight vaginal opening, and it hurt to try. Dismayed, I wrote to Ellen Barnard about how to stretch my vaginal entrance. Her advice to me (which follows) will be helpful to many of the women whose stories appear in this chapter.

Many of them report that they've gone without intercourse or other vaginal penetration for a long time. Then they meet someone who shivers their timbers, and they want to have vaginal sex again—but can't, due to pain.

An Expert Responds to Joan
ELLEN BARNARD, MSSW

Joan, it's not really about stretching the entrance to your vagina. It's more about how tight and how flexible the pelvic-floor muscles are at the opening of your vagina. After menopause, it gets more difficult for the pelvic floor to relax, unless you regularly practice doing so. Arousal helps with relaxation of the pelvic floor, thus allowing you to insert something inside your vagina comfortably. But after menopause it often takes a conscious relaxation effort, in addition to significant massage, for arousal.

So your task is to learn how to better relax those muscles, and to do so as you insert gradually wider toys. You are correct that you do need to work to accommodate something relatively similar in width to a penis if you hope to be engaging in intercourse again in the future. But don't "push" against those muscles—that doesn't work and actually causes them to tighten more. Instead, once you are fully aroused, gently slip a finger in alongside your favorite toy, taking a deep belly breath. Once you feel the opening relax, slip the finger a bit more inside. Instead of using a finger with a toy, you can use a tapered toy and insert it deeper as you breathe deeply and feel the vaginal opening relax.

RAE, AGE 61

How can I remedy the thinning of my vaginal walls so that sex is not painful? I haven't been sexual with a partner for about nine years. When I was about fifty-four, a very nice man and I got together, but we could not have sex vaginally. The pain was so great, I simply could not. It was like someone rubbing sandpaper inside me—not a turn-on for either partner.

It made me feel that a vibrant part of me wasn't there any longer. I thought I would be eighty or so before I had to think about changes in my sexuality in such a way. My ob-gyn told me it was the thinning of my vaginal walls, probably due to lack of estrogen. I used estrogen cream for a month or so but stopped, because I wasn't sexually active. I use a vibrator every three weeks or so. Strange thing is, I can still lubricate pretty well.

Recently an old lover and flame contacted me via Facebook, and we discovered there is still quite an attraction between us. We live in separate states and haven't set up any plans for a visit, but I know it will be happening soon. In the past, we had a very active sex life together. I have no idea what the outcome would be if I tried to have vaginal sex again.

He knows about this, and says all the right things, like, "There's plenty we can do without it being vaginal." However, having sex, especially vaginal sex, was what kept us so connected initially. I would hate to miss out on this opportunity to see what we might rediscover with one another, but I'm feeling very anxious about planning a trip to see him.

I fear not being able to have vaginal sex, because unless this gets managed somehow, there is no way it can happen.

An Expert Responds

ELLEN BARNARD, MSSW

It's a shock when we discover that something that was once so pleasurable now hurts. Many women are having this experience, because they have not been actively engaging in consistent vaginal penetration—which is two to three times per week—to maintain good vaginal health. Here's what you can do to get yourself to a place where you can enjoy vaginal penetration during sex:

- Start with our Vaginal Renewal program,[1] which will moisturize the vaginal skin. Even though you are lubricating—which is a sign of excellent overall physical health—you may still be quite dry at times other than during sexual arousal. This program will bring blood flow into the vaginal skin cells and will build up the skin and the layers beneath it. Do both external and internal massage every day at first, until you notice that the skin is becoming thicker and more flexible. Then continue at two to three times a week to maintain good vaginal health. Vaginal massage does not have to result in arousal—it can just be done as a therapeutic activity and doesn't have to lead to any other sexual activity. It's really just a daily internal massage to keep the skin healthy.

- You can choose to pair this program with the short-term use of estrogen gel or the Estring (estrogen ring), which will speed up the time it takes to restore the skin's flexibility and thickness. (We don't like the estrogen cream, because it contains oils that can break down condoms and irritate the vaginal skin.)

- Enjoy orgasms once or twice a week; this helps keep the nerves functioning well and encourages more frequent lubrication.

- Exercise your pelvic-floor muscles by doing Kegels, paying equal attention to the contraction *and* the relaxation of the muscles that surround the vagina in particular. Otherwise you may find that these muscles are stiff and inflexible, which will also get in the way of comfortable penetration when you are ready to have it.

If you find that penetration hurts with a sharp pain, or if it feels like there is a stiff ring at the opening that you can't get past easily, get a referral for a pelvic-floor therapist to help you relax those muscles again. Then you can learn how to control their tension and relaxation so that you can enjoy penetration fully.

You will be ready for intercourse when you can comfortably fit three of your fingers inside your vagina once you are aroused. When you are planning on having intercourse, I recommend you use a silicone-based lubricant, which protects your skin more than a water-based lubricant and is compatible with condoms.

Don't despair! This can be addressed with some attention and a bit of work every day. In the meantime, if you get together with this old flame, I hope you will choose to enjoy the wonderful variety of intimate pleasures available to the two of you until you're ready to explore intercourse.

ADVICE FROM AN EXPERT
Vulvar/Vaginal Irritation?
BY SUSAN KELLOGG SPADT, PHD, CRNP

Many common products—several that may surprise you—can irritate your vulva and vagina. Try eliminating these:

- minipads, particularly scented ones, with strong adhesive and/or "wings"

- shampoo/conditioner used on pubic hair

- dryer sheets/fabric softeners, particularly when used on underclothing

- douches (the vagina is self-cleaning with its own fluid, no need to cleanse it internally)

- benzyl alcohol (a preservative in many vaginal creams, cleansers, shampoos, and fragrances)

➤

- glycerin (an ingredient in many lubricants; instead try organic products such as Good Clean Love, www .goodcleanlove.com, for highly sensitive, allergic skin)

- shaving cream for legs—don't use it to shave genitals

- any genital product that says it "warms" or "cools" the skin

- diets high in sugar

OLIVIA, AGE 69

My husband is one sweet man, appreciative and enthusiastic. He has the desire, the ability, and the stamina to truly satisfy me. I love to bury my face in the hair on his chest. I love its smell and feel. I love his hands on my body. I love his legs. I love his laugh.

My only difficulty has been dryness and a constriction in my vaginal opening. Once my husband began Viagra and I quit taking hormones, it became impossible to have penetration. I wish it were otherwise, but we both are able to have orgasms with stimulation from our hands and mouths. The arousal to desire continues as before: kissing, sharing poems (especially erotic ones), soft music, touching, and fondling each other.

When I first began having problems, I was embarrassed during a pap smear, because it hurt. My gynecologist sent me to a physical therapist, who did some vaginal-stretching exercises. I was relieved when a possible solution was posed. But when we didn't have regular penetrative sex and I didn't keep up the stretching, my vaginal opening shrank again. Bleeding continued throughout the stretching the therapist did, and I eventually lost hope of real improvement.

Joan Responds

Olivia, you clearly love your husband and the intimacy between you, even though it doesn't include penetration right now. You don't need to give up on penetration, though. Please resume doing the exercises you learned from the pelvic-floor physical therapist, and add the other parts of the Vaginal Renewal program that Ellen Barnard and Myrtle Wilhite describe in this chapter, such as the Kegel relaxations and the vaginal massage. You can do the vaginal massage on your own, or enlist your loving husband to help you, your choice!

LAUREN, AGE 61

Recently I had sex for the first time in twelve years. Apparently one's vagina does change after not using it for a long period of time. I always thought sex was like riding a bicycle, but one can't just get back on and ride! I experienced such pain during the attempted penetration that we had to stop. What a disappointing and embarrassing moment. My partner was very understanding. I was frustrated and disappointed.

I went to my gynecologist for an examination and explained my circumstances. She gave me a thorough exam and said that although I had many tiny lacerations and redness, my vagina seemed normal. She explained how one's vaginal lining becomes thin after menopause, and her advice was to abstain from sex for two weeks, using lubrication to aid in healing.

When we engaged in sex again, very gently, I was once again disappointed with the level of pain, even with lots of lubrication. We once again had to stop. So now I am wondering if there is some way I can stretch my vagina, for it seems like it has shrunk. Perhaps it is just my imagination running wild? Is there a solution? For your information, I have never been on hormones, and my partner's penis is of normal size.

Joan Responds

Lauren, take a look at Ellen's response to my concerns, at the beginning of this section. I think her response to me could be very helpful to your situation.

MELANIA, AGE 70

I have overcome many issues in life—changing from the conservative religion of my parents and giving up the sexual inhibitions of younger days. Okay, I spent a few bucks and lots of therapy time to evolve. I *love* that my past three marriages have given me a richness and complexity that allows me the freedom to go for the gold. I am very secure in my sexuality, in the knowledge that I have the ability to deeply care for a special man in my life, and that I can satisfy and be satisfied. What more could I ask for than that?

My third husband had Alzheimer's. He could barely perform, but I loved him dearly. I adjusted to what he had, and I could usually be orgasmic with any stimulation. Now, after one divorce and the death of two husbands, I am two months into a new relationship: a man six years my junior whose wife died of cancer.

We are both in the same situation. Our beloved spouses are dead. We are both the living remains of two good marriages. We both had been celibate during our spouses' illnesses (during the end of cancer and Alzheimer's, there's no marriage bed) and after their deaths.

As my anticipation of a potential sexual partner started the juices flowing, I was aware of vaginal stinging. I explained to a pharmacist "no discharge, no odor, no itch," and she pointed me to lubricants and a gave me a "not to worry" approach.

After a husband with illness and flaccidity, I have a virile man in my life! Our first attempt at intimacy, though, was painful, even though I thought I was doing enough self-pleasure with a vibrator to be in shape. The pain of my first sexual penetration with my new lover shocked me.

I made an appointment with my general practitioner. He assured me nothing was wrong and that I should just try to find a comfortable position. At that point, I ordered *Better Than I Ever Expected* and did the Vaginal Renewal plan daily, and apparently it worked. I was prepared to have to wait a month or two, but after ten days, I was "good to go" the next time we were together. We had a week of terrific sex!

I am loving the surprise of a delicious man in my life. He is a kind man—thanks me for every meal I prepare, even puts the toilet seat down. We talk about *everything*—he says he has never had a woman as open as I am. He has been understanding and totally available for sex as I adjust to having a penis in my life!

Sex is wonderful but so is just sharing the bed with someone I am caring for more every day. We come to each other with a deep and complex past and have a future in which to share and grow.

Note from Joan: The following steps on how to massage and renew your vagina originally appeared in *Better Than I Ever Expected*, where Dr. Wilhite's tips for perfect Kegels also appear.

ADVICE FROM AN EXPERT

Tips for Vaginal Health

BY MYRTLE WILHITE, MD

External Moisturizing and Massage

Increase the suppleness and blood circulation of the skin of your vulva and vagina with a five- to ten-minute massage using a moisturizing sexual lubricant like Liquid Silk. Liquid Silk is a water-based lotion that will soak in and moisturize your skin; it won't get sticky and will help you massage with very little friction.

Push in to the skin with circular strokes, and massage what's underneath the skin, rather than brushing across the skin. Include the inner lips, the hood of the clitoris, the head of the clitoris, and the perineum.

To complete your external massage, massage into the opening of the vaginal canal, using the same circular strokes. The massage itself does not need to be self-sexual in any way, but if that is comfortable for you, by all means, explore these sensations.

Internal Vaginal Massage

To massage inside your vaginal canal, we suggest using a dildo made of Lucite, which is very smooth and will not cause friction

➤

or tearing. Choose your size based upon how many fingers you can comfortably insert into the opening of your vagina.

After a session of external vulva massage, apply the same massage to the inner surfaces of your vagina with your dildo (with lubricant applied on both skin and dildo). Rather than pushing the dildo in and out, use a circular massage movement. You are increasing skin flexibility so that your body can adjust to comfortable sexual penetration if you choose it.

You might also choose to use a slim vibrator for massaging the vaginal walls. Coat it in Liquid Silk, and then insert it gently. Turn it on and let it run for about five minutes. You don't need to move it around; just lie there and let it do its work.

Orgasm

Be aware that if you're not having orgasms, the blood vessels can literally get out of shape, preventing future orgasms. If you are able to bring yourself to orgasm, do so at least once a week—for the rest of your life. (Seriously.) This is preventive maintenance of your body.

Kegel Relaxation

Kegels increase both the strength and flexibility of your pelvic-floor muscles. Pay attention to the relaxation and deep-breath part of the exercise. Learning to relax your pelvic floor will help you to avoid tensing up before penetration.

When Doctors Don't Help

Doctors get almost no training in sexuality, and unless they make this a priority in their education and practice, you might need to ask for a referral to a specialist. Otherwise, you may have experiences like Martha's (see below). Our medical professionals have to understand that we value our genital health and want sexual pleasure for the rest of our lives. Sometimes they go after information on their own, like a dedicated gynecologist I know who bought two dozen copies of *Better Than I Ever Expected* to give to her older patients. (I hope she'll do that with this book too.) If our doctors aren't making the effort, maybe we can start to educate them ourselves, as Esther chose to do (see below).

MARTHA, AGE 65

Why does it hurt to have intercourse? Why can't I fix it? Do not tell me I have an infection, and do not prescribe antibiotics—that is *not* what's wrong.

I've seen a gynecologist several times, even though it hurts to have the speculum inserted. Each new gynecologist prescribed antibiotics, though there was absolutely no sign of infection. I went back for follow-up to be told, each and every time, "Well, there's still no evidence of infection; if the pain still exists, it must be something else. I don't know what." Finally I just gave up.

One male gynecologist said, "You can't be feeling pain. You have no nerve endings there." I should have reached over, squeezed his balls hard, and told him, "You can't be feeling pain. You have no nerve endings there."

I connected with my second husband when I was forty. We actively worked at giving each other the best sex of our lives. We had great, mind-blowing sex for years. In my late forties I started not wanting it every day and started having difficulty reaching orgasm. My husband was understanding and patient—and also loved to give head, as did I. So we often did not have full intercourse.

In my midfifties, I started having pain during intercourse. At first it was just when he'd enter me—although he was always gentle and made sure I was lubricated. Later it hurt with every stroke. I became less interested in intercourse and in sex generally. I tried for a few years to make up for it by giving him head, but eventually that became a chore for me.

Finally we had no sex at all for five years. I thought he was okay with it. But then I discovered he was having an affair with a seventeen-year-old girl (he was forty-eight), and then with a close gay male friend. I didn't want to lose him and was very jealous, so I seduced him, and we started having regular sex again. I said nothing of my pain to him, but he watched my face closely as he entered me, and I think he knew. Still, for the next few years, we had sex once or twice a week.

In my early sixties, I just didn't feel like it at all anymore, and he was okay with that. Then he got very sick, and he died within two years. When he was first diagnosed, he asked for and got the best blow job of his life; then never was interested again, nor was I.

After he died, I had a dream where we were having sex, and I awoke with an intense orgasm. Since then, about once a month, I feel the urge and masturbate to mind-blowing orgasm. As I don't intend to have intercourse again, the pain actually is no longer a problem for me. I suppose I'm going to be celibate all the rest of my life. I am making my peace with this. Ah well.

Joan Responds

Martha, you're too young to decide you'll never have inter-course again. I hope you'll keep yourself open emotionally and physically. I suspect you're still in mourning and not ready to make any decisions about future relationships. It's wonderful that you can experience mind-blowing orgasms on your own. For your sexual health, once a week would be better than once a month, so I hope you'll consider pleasuring yourself, even when you don't feel the urge—the arousal will come!

ESTHER, AGE 63

In my early forties, I needed more lubrication and didn't know that the K-Y Jelly recommended by my doctor was giving me yeast infections. I assumed it was my late husband. Every time we had sex, I got a yeast infection—which took two to three weeks to clear up, as my physician refused to give me a pre-scription, leaving me to guess about over-the-counter prod-ucts. This took the happy anticipation out of intercourse. Sex slowly exited my life, and now, fifteen years later, I'm dealing with diminished vaginal-tissue elasticity.

I asked my doctor to help, and she prescribed estrogen cream. I'm also using the Vaginal Renewal program suggested on the Woman's Touch website (www.a-womans-touch.com). I sure hope it improves things so I can tolerate penetration once again. Fortunately, my partner is understanding and patient, and we have discovered many other ways to pleasure and sat-isfy each other. I worry about permanent loss of the ability to experience and enjoy vaginal penetration.

I felt that my doctor—though she's a woman just a few years younger that I—was not totally comfortable going beyond the simple suggestions of hormone-replacement cream. I'm getting bolder in my old age, and I opened a discussion of sex after sixty, giving her a list of websites and books that I had found helpful. I told her I thought they might be helpful in counseling her ever-growing number of patients having to deal with becoming sexually active after years of no sex.

Interestingly, when I went back to see my doctor, she said, "I had the opportunity to share the information you gave me with some other patients."

Vulvar/Vaginal Pain Resources

Vulvar/vaginal pain is a complex issue. I hope that this chapter gave you some information and direction for getting your pain diagnosed and treated. These websites offer more information and/or referrals to knowledgeable professionals:

- American Association of Sexuality Educators, Counselors, and Therapists: www.aasect.org

- American Physical Therapist Association, Section on Women's Health: www.womenshealthapta.org

- American Urogynecologic Society: www.augs.org

- International Society for the Study of Vulvar Disease: www.issvd.org

- Mypelvichealth.org: www.mypelvichealth.org

- National Vulvodynia Association: www.nva.org

- Obgyn.net: www.obgyn.net

- Pelvic and Sexual Health Institute: www.pelvicand sexualhealthinstitute.org

- Secret Suffering, Helping Women Cope with Sexual and Pelvic Pain: www.secretsuffering.com

- Vulval Pain Society: www.vulvalpainsociety.org

- Vulvar Pain Foundation: www.vulvarpain foundation.org

- Vulvodynia.com: www.vulvodynia.com

Note: You can find this list with hyperlinks for your convenience at www.NakedAtOurAge.com.

12

Reclaiming Sexuality after Cancer

WHEN ROBERT WAS recovering from his chemotherapy, as sick and exhausted as he felt, it was important to him to touch and be touched. As soon as he was able, he wanted to make love. But we wondered if it was safe for me. Would the chemicals in his system be in his ejaculate, and if so, would that affect me? Should we use a condom?

The infusion center had sent Robert home with a big folder packed with information. It covered everything he might need to know, except for one glaring omission: There was no mention of sex whatsoever.

Robert phoned the infusion center to ask. The nurse seemed stunned that sex could be on his mind, as sick and beaten down as people feel after chemo. She did answer the question: We should wait a week or so, then it should be safe. (I learned later that this varies with the actual drugs used, so don't go by our experience.) But we got the impression that it never occurred to them that patients would want to know this—and that patients never asked.

It wasn't a physical urge that drove Robert—his physical urges were only to sleep and try to eat. But for him—always an intensely physical person—reclaiming his sexuality was an *emotional* imperative, a way to affirm that he was fully alive, and that his body was capable of pleasure, not just disease and treatments. For us as a couple, bonding sexually was an exhilarating assertion that we could get past the emotional trauma of his cancer, the invasive treatment that left him weak and sick, and the fear that he would die.

I'm crying as I write this, because Robert did die—but more than two years later. The chemo gave him two more years to regain his health, create stunning art (see www.robertriceart .com), dance, and live fully—including sexually. We got married during that time. I'm grateful beyond words.

What to Expect

In this section, you'll find lots of practical advice for working around the sex-related problems that accompany cancer. I hope these stories and this expert advice will be helpful and enhance your intimacy.

MAGGIE, AGE 62

Recently, I started dating a nice guy who had surgery for prostate cancer seven months ago. He told me all the bad news that the doctor had told him about side effects. He advised me that he would never be able to have an ejaculation, and that sex for him would never be the same. I got the idea that he would never feel the pleasure of having a climax again. My fear is that if this is true, what would be the point of him having sex? Where can I get some straight answers on what we are looking at, possibility-wise? I am a very sexual woman and would just like to know if there is any chance that there can be a sexual relationship.

An Expert Responds

ANNE KATZ, RN, PHD

There are a number of possibilities in this situation, some of them good, and some of them not so good. Here are the facts.

Surgery for prostate cancer (a radical prostatectomy, or complete removal of the prostate gland) will result in significant changes in a man's ability to have an erection. Depending on what his erections were like before the surgery, and the amount of damage that the surgery has done to the nerves responsible for erections, the man may be able to have erections after the surgery. But he most likely will always need help from medications like Viagra, Cialis, or Levitra. These medications only help about 50 percent of the time for men who take them after treatment for prostate cancer, but other erectile aids, such as the vacuum pump or penile injections, can help too.

Some men are able to have an erection, but it may not last very long. Some men can only achieve a thickening of the penis that may not be sufficient for penetration. Progress in regaining erections may continue for up to two years after surgery, and what he has at that point is usually as good as it is going to get.

Orgasms are still possible, even with a flaccid penis. The orgasm will not be accompanied by ejaculation (the prostate gland makes the fluid portion of the ejaculate, and so when it is gone, so is the emission). Some men report more intense orgasms after this surgery; some say they are much less intense.

Libido (sexual desire) is not affected by removal of the prostate, but the mind is a very important part of a man's sexuality. Repeated failure to have an erection sufficient for penetration may cause him to lose some interest.

Many couples find a way around these difficulties. There are more ways than just penetration for both the man and the woman to achieve orgasm and satisfaction, and some creativity goes a long way. This may be challenging for a new relationship. But the lust and attraction in a new relationship may also provide extra impetus.

This is a couple's issue, and both partners have to work on finding a solution. Communication is a very important part of sexuality. Talk openly about what works for him and what doesn't, what you want, and what creativity you can both bring to sexual activity.

ADVICE FROM AN EXPERT
Sex and Intimacy after Cancer
BY SAGE BOLTE, PHD, MSW, LCSW, OSW-C

Sexuality is a critical part of your quality of life. Sex and intimacy are key ways to affirm "I'm alive, I'm human," and to get back what was important to you before cancer.

Cancer and its treatment may change sexual function, which can impact your willingness to engage in sexual activity. However, patience and willingness to learn new techniques can help you regain a positive sense of sexual confidence.

Here are tips for coping with some specific problems.

- Vaginal dryness and discomfort: Apply 100 percent vitamin E oil to the vaginal tissues and clitoris on a regular basis after showering (not during sex); this helps with the dryness and is good for the general

➤

health of the vaginal tissue. Then use a water-based lubricant as needed during sex. Talk to your doctor about whether an estrogen ring or testosterone patch would be appropriate to regain vaginal moisture and elasticity. After radiation to the pelvis, some women find that inserting plain yogurt into the vagina with fingers or a dilator helps with comfort and pH balance. If you have pain with sex that is not resolved with increased lubrication, you may be experiencing vaginal stenosis (the narrowing of the vaginal canal), vaginal atrophy, or another problem that should be addressed with your gynecologist. Your healthcare provider may recommend dilator therapy to treat and manage vaginal pain/discomfort.

- Erectile dysfunction: Tell your physician about this, and find out if your medications are exacerbating the problem. Check your testosterone levels. If you're having a harder time maintaining an erection, find the position that is most stimulating for you. Help your partner reach orgasm before intercourse. Devices for men that may help include penile pumps, injections, suppositories, implants, or rings. Always discuss options with your physician first: If you're on blood thinners or have low platelets, these devices might put you at risk. Viagra and similar medications are not recommended for men who have heart concerns or who are taking blood-pressure medication.

- Pain and fatigue: After cancer treatment, the time of day that's best for sex might change. If you're exhausted in the evening, switch to morning or afternoon. Take pain medication thirty to sixty minutes before sexual activity. Get exercise, which can minimize fatigue and decrease some joint pain. A warm bath or shower can also help reduce pain and can be a pleasurable starting place for your sexual play. Rest during sex—it's not a marathon.

- Fear of rejection: Consider seeing a couples' counselor or sex therapist. Often the problems of miscommunication, misinterpretation, and anxiety get in the way of your sexuality and intimacy. Realize that if you had problems in your relationship prior to cancer, those issues do not disappear and will resurface; they need to be addressed.

- Difficulties reconnecting with your partner: Communicate your desires, ask for what you need, and ask your partner to communicate honestly too. Make time to be together and to connect. Be affectionate in a relaxed way—hold hands, make eye contact, touch gently, kiss, massage each other. Take it slow and easy. If your partner is not interested in sexual play, you can find ways to please yourself. If your partner is afraid of hurting you or has other questions, speak to the doctor together about these concerns.

- Difficulties getting stimulated or aroused: Take more time. Instead of the physiological response coming first and driving the emotional response, it may need to be the other way around—a mind thing first. Spend

➤

time reflecting, planning, and reminding yourself how it felt to be aroused. Schedule your sex time: thinking about it, fantasizing, and working yourself up to mental excitement will stimulate the physical excitement. Don't let sex feel like pressure to perform. Sometimes you can practice just touching without the expectation of intercourse. Start with self-pleasuring experiences. Your body has changed since your diagnosis and treatment. You need to become comfortable touching yourself and knowing what feels good now in order to show your partner what feels good.

Sometimes you can't get back to the sexual function you had prior to cancer, but that doesn't mean it can't be good or pleasurable. Focus on touch, sensation, and pleasurable feelings. Use sex toys. Engage in mutual masturbation. Read fantasy to each other. Touch yourself. Massage each other and cuddle. Being naked and cuddling is a powerfully intimate and sensual act.

Sometimes You Have to Laugh

As frightened as BillyBob was about his prostate cancer testing and treatment, his sense of humor served him well:

BILLYBOB, AGE 62

I complained to my doctor that I was constantly peeing. He did the up-the-butt routine which we all hate so much. He recommended I see a urologist for a prostate test. The day I was supposed to have this test, the equipment was down, but the doctor said he had this sales lady for new equipment he was thinking of buying. He asked if I would be willing to let this strange lady do the testing. I agreed. It felt kind of funny having a lady put a probe up my butt. The test was like a seminar, her doing the testing, and explaining how the equipment worked to the doctor. It kind of felt like a three-ring circus—and I was the clown.

The test was not bad, but the results sure were. They found I had prostate cancer. I was floored—my brain was about to have a blooming fit.

The treatment by radiation was painless except for my pride—I had to be naked and seen by whichever nurse tech was handling the daily treatments for eight weeks at twelve seconds a shot. I made a game out of it to help with the embarrassment. I bought fake tattoos and placed one every day in the appropriate area. The nurse techs enjoyed seeing what one I had on for that day. So there was some laughter almost every session, and that eased my personal pain.

GERALD, AGE 73

A seventyish man who was recovering from a prostatectomy asked fellow members of a prostate-cancer support group how they could have sex if they were leaking urine. He ended with, "My wife is willing to be pissed off but not pissed on."

Despite the laughter, his was a serious problem. The first response solved it: "Put a band on your penis—a cock ring. A lot of older guys who aren't incontinent use them to maintain erections, but if you're leaking, they're a good answer, especially if you use a pump."

The first man admitted, "I hadn't thought of that. We've never used any . . . devices. Of course, I've never had prostate cancer before, either." The prostate-cancer world introduces many guys to devices and positions and concepts previously unimagined.

I was rendered impotent by prostate surgery and radiation. A physician pal told me, "You'd better start pumping up your penis every day, whether you're going to use it or not, or it'll shrivel into a Vienna sausage. As soon as you lose spontaneous erections, you lose penile tone. No tone, and there'll be nothing to pump when you do want to use it."

Sex is the second-most common topic—after cancer therapies—at most prostate-cancer support groups. Many men—impotent and perhaps stripped of libido by hormonal ablation—simply but not happily accept the verdict that their sex lives are over. This is grave, since sexuality can represent the life force's most powerful affirmation in the face of death. I think that making love as long as one can and as well as one can represents life refusing to give in to death or infirmity.

Unfortunately, many of us men grow up believing that our sexuality dwells almost exclusively in our genitals, so a damaged penis may lead to a damaged personality. As one wife admitted at a session for couples, "There's not much fun in our lives anymore, and I don't just mean sex. He's just so sad." A penile fixation may also lead us to forget how much sexual satisfaction can be achieved by giving pleasure to a partner we love.

I addressed such issues directly in my novel *Grace Period*, because so many people seem to have misinformation or no information about the relationship of sex to illness and aging. In the novel, I tell the story of two cancer survivors who are in their sixties when they meet. Both have been physically damaged by their illnesses: Marty is impotent and suffers from urinary incontinence, while Miranda has endured a mastectomy and wonders if she can ever be attractive again. They become lovers.

Marty and Miranda consider sex a natural expression of their love, so they pursue it creatively and with gentle persistence. They discover an L position for intercourse that allows some penetration, even without an erection; and when Miranda falls too ill for sexual intercourse, they enjoy the shared pleasure of Marty washing her hair.

In my view, sex is too important a part of loving relationships to give up easily. Marty and Miranda compensate for physical deficiencies with their inventiveness and passion. Well past libidinous youth, those two remain profoundly sensual. They never lose love and concern for one another, and every touch becomes precious, a kind of grace.

—Gerald Haslam, who is living with prostate cancer, is the author of eighteen books (including Grace Period, *a novel about prostate cancer) and the editor of eight anthologies. You can visit his website at www.geraldhaslam.com.*

NEIL, AGE 74

A diagnosis of cancer is very frightening. For me, the journey was scary enough without the myths and misinformation I was told about cancer of the prostate.

"After age fifty-five, sex doesn't matter that much anyway," a physician who specializes in the treatment of prostate cancer told me. He believed his words would be comforting. They weren't! I promised the doctor that I would look him up on his fifty-fifth birthday and tell him to "cut that out." He sheepishly smiled and said, "Oh my. I think I said something wrong."

We often are not told that the penis will be about an inch shorter after surgery. Because the urethra passes through the prostate, when the prostate is removed, that portion of the urethra is removed as well. Then, when the urethra is resectioned, the penis is drawn in toward the abdomen. Secure circumcised males seem able to weather this storm, but uncircumcised males have an additional problem. The surgery leaves more foreskin than before. This additional tissue traps urine and produces odor. Baby wipes do a fine job of solving this problem.

The missionary position is usually no longer successful after prostate surgery. The prostate stabilizes the penis and prevents it from receding into the abdominal cavity, so removal of the prostate decreases penile stability. The angle of the vagina, coupled with a shortened penis with no internal stability, means missionary style may not work. I found, however, that doggie style, "side by side," and "woman on top" work just fine.

I must warn about the product advertisements that flood the market about penile enhancement, instant erections, and so on. Some of these can be harmful to a cancer survivor. Some are loaded with testosterone, which can cause further growth of prostate cancer. Check with your physician before trying any medications.

I am blessed with a caring and competent urologist (not the one who said sex doesn't matter!) who has given me nine years free of prostate cancer. The urologist was aggressive in treatment and caught the disease early. My physician candidly stated that doctors don't get much training in sexuality. When faced with a choice of saving my life or providing me with sex education, I would want my doctor to go after the cancer. I am here today because of this priority. Men should find a competent urologist and stay with their professional judgment. This stuff is nothing to mess with or take lightly.

At all times, we need to keep our partners involved in the options we're considering. They can be our most precious friends and supporters. They deserve to be part of the solution to our new life experiences.

EVONNE, AGE 58

My fiancé (age sixty-eight) and I are in an incredible, sensual, passionate relationship. We met about a year ago. Sparks flew immediately, and we jumped full force into each other, emotionally. I was quite surprised—I didn't know I could be that passionate again, and neither did he. My new lover aroused me in ways I never felt before. What a ride!

My lover has had prostate cancer, and so we didn't expect much sexually. He is not able to sustain an erection. But what the man can do with his hands! He is able to give me "inside" orgasms as well as out. All I can say is "endless foreplay and multiple orgasms." We play for at least an hour. At first, it was a little weird to kiss and caress him while he was not erect. But I got over it, and we both get so much pleasure out of it.

We are enjoying being truly desired. I am slightly overweight and always felt uncomfortable about my body with my ex-husband. But my new lover tells me often how much he loves every inch of me. What a gift to my self-esteem he has been!

We sleep in the nude, which greatly enhances our activity, as we are always open and available to each other's touch, and arousal usually follows. Cuddling is a great source of comfort and intimacy for us. We are both in shock over the pleasure this sexual relationship gives us. We are in love, and I truly believe that we could only reach this level of connection and intimacy in a spiritually committed relationship. We are getting married in June.

LOLA, AGE 71

I shudder at the mere thought of a first date. What if your belly lops over, and your chest is flat because you donated two breasts to cancer? I had a bilateral mastectomy without reconstruction. I never thought it would make a difference.

However, I decided to flirt with an older man I know from my volunteer work. This man knows I've had breast cancer. It started out as a fun mental diversion for me, and I suggested we have a date. I never thought he would take the bait, but he did, and now I'm petrified that things may develop into a sexual encounter.

I may be jumping the gun by worrying about such a stupid thing. I have always had body-image problems, because I'm chubby and have a big butt and fat legs—which look worse with no boobs. Oh, woe is me!

I left my marriage in 1988 after twenty-four years and really had no interest in dating until I met this man. I feel like a stupid teenager. Besides the issue about the boobs, what is worse is this: What if you have to fart, or worse yet, fart in bed?

I really don't think this man is judgmental about body image—he can't be any great shakes himself, since he is eighty-three. But I'm having a horrible time getting past the issues of no boobs, fat butt and legs, and farting.

Joan Responds

Lola, go for it! If you've already told him about your breast cancer—and he's eighty-three himself—I can't imagine that either of you will be expecting each other's body to look perfect . . . or to work perfectly, for that matter.

You don't have to jump into bed the first hour of your first date. You could spend the first date just having fun together, with clothes on, and getting to know each other. It will only serve to increase the anticipation for the second date, and whatever might happen then. During your face-to-face conversation, it would be honest and helpful to tell him that you had a double mastectomy, and that you're interested in a sexual relationship, and that you're nervous as hell. He may have some things to share himself!

As for the fear of farting (and I find it hilarious that you think that's scarier than sharing your body-image concerns), I actually do have some advice.

- Have sex before dinner instead of afterward.

- For a whole day before your date, don't eat any of the foods that give you gas.

- If you fart in bed, laugh and say, "Was that you? Don't worry, it's okay!"

An Update on Lola

Lola wrote again after her date.

"Well, Lola got what she wanted! Three nights and two days with a wonderful man. I didn't fart—he did! We both laughed so hard about handling "the first fart." Not having any boobs wasn't such a big issue. Turned out he had issues of his own related to prostate surgery. Lots of hugging and kissing and cuddling, and it turned out to be everything I could have hoped for in my first date in eighteen years. The whole situation was a gift to me, as I was able to step so far out of my comfort zone. So there you have it!"

Sex and Healing

Especially when you're with a loving partner, sex can be a strong part of the healing process, as you'll see in these stories.

DOUG, AGE 65

When I was forty-four, I was diagnosed with acute leukemia. I was near death when I arrived at the hospital. I underwent three courses of aggressive chemotherapy over four months. I lost my hair, had pneumonia three times, and almost died. I cannot remember having any interest in sex.

Slowly I got better and stronger, and the urge for sex returned. Being a cancer survivor provided its own set of challenges in living my life and in my sexuality. The ability to make love to my wife helped in my healing, both physically and emotionally.

A year ago, I needed quadruple heart bypass surgery. The rehab program was long and difficult. I had no strength or appetite, could not sleep, and was haunted by my own fragile mortality. Sex was not part of the process at first.

My wife knows me better than I know myself. Without her, I could not have gotten back on my feet to where I am today, physically and emotionally. Sex became part of the healing process. When the feelings to become sexually intimate again emerged, I worried that the excitement and physical exertion might be troublesome for my repaired heart. We made adjustments to our love life.

We purchased a vibrator, though my wife was hesitant. When she finally tried it, it was an instant hit. She had orgasms like never before: strong and multiples. I was excited that she was so satisfied with our modified sex.

She felt guilty that she was getting the satisfaction with our new techniques, so she asked what she could do to increase my pleasure. I asked if she would let me watch her pleasure herself, and if she would watch me do the same to myself. We opened new horizons to pleasure through self-pleasuring.

We have normal intercourse on occasion, but frankly, the use of the vibrator and self-pleasuring is much more satisfying. My wife has found my G-spot under my scrotum, and she massages it while I masturbate until I get a tremendous orgasm. An orgasm in this fashion beats any that I get via penetration sex.

We never lose our need for sexual satisfaction. It seems to me that sex is more fulfilling in later years than when we are younger, because both partners are more mature and experienced. We know better how to please one another.

CLARK, AGE 58

I was diagnosed with multiple myeloma—cancer of the bone marrow—when I was fifty-one. I thought my life was coming to an end. I have fought diligently to stay alive. I had my first stem-cell transplant and was told there was a 5 to 10 percent chance I would not survive it, as it wreaks havoc on your body and heart. I made it, but some others who were in the same hospital did not. I was a very sick puppy, as I was also receiving high doses of chemotherapy.

I had five different chemotherapies and two stem-cell transplants over six and a half years. My doctors said that I almost or could have died five out of the six times I was in the hospital.

My libido went to zero for five years, starting with my cancer diagnosis. I felt distraught thinking my libido and sexual feelings would never return. Feeling sexual is very important to me and always has been, since the age of ten. I tried to masturbate, but I ended up with painful muscle spasms in my stomach. It actually hurt. Then, about a year ago, my libido started to return. It felt wonderful. I started researching sexuality, attending workshops about cancer and intimacy, and watching sex-ed videos like those at www.sexsmartfilms.com, which is run by sexologist, Mark Schoen, PhD.

I wake up every morning with fatigue and pain due to a compression fracture in my spine and the cancer treatment.

But to be honest, I have never felt so sexual as I do now. To me, that's a great thing.

MILES, AGE 64

The day we found out I had prostate cancer was terrible. When we got home, we decided to give each other a long hug every day. It's easy to forget things like that. We also decided that we would call going to bed together "play time," and not have the expectation of sex, so there would be less disappointment if there were difficulties.

I chose IMRT treatment. Before and during the treatment, I was given monthly Lupron shots to stop the production of testosterone. Yes, it is possible to have sex without testosterone, but it is more difficult. During the Lupron, my wife and I managed to have a sexual encounter once a week. It wasn't nearly as good as before, but it was still wonderful. A dedicated and loving partner makes all the difference.

Now I am off the Lupron, and our sex life is nearly back to where it was before all this. A loving wife and a little Levitra can do wonders. We make love about twice a week now. I am sometimes pretty tired at night, but "nooners" can be real fun.

I would like men and women to know that there can be sex after prostate cancer. Choose your doctors and treatments wisely, and love each other with all your being. Prostate cancer is a terrible thing, but it is not the end of a loving relationship.

The Importance of Talking

With a cancer diagnosis, life goes into overdrive. There are so many medical, emotional, and daily-life concerns, and with all the fear, it's hard to stay focused. But especially if you're in a committed relationship, it's important to make sure sexual intimacy doesn't fall off the radar.

Psychologist and sex therapist Stephanie Buehler sees many people with chronic illness. She offers these tips for bringing sex back into your life after cancer, a heart attack, or other major illnesses.

ADVICE FROM AN EXPERT
Reclaiming Sexuality after a Health Event
BY STEPHANIE BUEHLER, PSYD

No question, a major illness can leave your sexuality bruised. But you can learn how to be sexual with one another despite changes or limitations. Your sex life may not be the same, but it can still be satisfying.

- Speak to your physician about when you can resume sex, and what kinds of limitations you might expect or need to work around. If you are uncomfortable talking about it with the physician, bring it up to the nurse. Nurses are trained to educate patients and are interested in helping them achieve an optimal quality of life.

- If neither the physician nor the nurse is sexually savvy, contact the organization associated with your disease. For example, both the American Heart Association and the American Cancer Society publish booklets on sexuality and illness.

- Broaden your ideas about what constitutes sex after an illness event. Sex is more than intercourse. Count

➤

➤

cuddling as sex, and you and your partner might feel less disappointed or glum.

- If you are the person affected with a health problem, don't conclude that if your partner isn't bringing up sex, it is no longer important. Your partner may not want to intrude or make demands, and may be waiting for a sign of readiness from you.

- If you are the partner of the person with a health problem, go together to a physician's visit to discuss the possible sexual effects of any surgery or treatment. Educate yourself so that you can be a support to your partner, and so that you both can discuss how to go forward.

- If you had sexual problems before the illness event, address them with your physician or nurse. It may be that your health problem contributed to your sexual problem.

- If you are having trouble resuming satisfying sexual activity, a sex therapist can help you identify obstacles, give you information and suggestions, and address deeper problems.

Advice from the National Cancer Institute

Even for a couple that has been together a long time, staying connected can be a major challenge at first. It may be comforting to learn that very few committed relationships end because of ostomies, scars, or other body changes. Divorce rates are about the same for people with and without a cancer history.

Tell your partner how you feel about your sex life and what you would like to change. You might want to talk about your concerns, your beliefs about why your sex life is the way it is, your feelings, and what would make you feel better. Approaching it openly avoids blame, stays positive, and gives your partner a better sense of how you are feeling. Here is an example of how you might start your discussion: "I know it's tough to talk about, but I think we should discuss our sex life. We've only made love a few times lately. I miss being close to you. I worry that my scars might be a problem. Can you tell me how you feel?"

Try to be open-minded as you listen to your partner's point of view:

- Focus on your partner's comments, not on what you plan to say in response.

- Repeat what he or she says in your own words.

- Ask questions to better understand your partner's concerns.

- Acknowledge that your partner's views matter to you. Say things like "I see why you might think that" or "I never thought of it that way before."

—National Cancer Institute, www.cancer.gov, offers information for cancer patients and their families.[1]

Learning Acceptance

Clearly it's easier to deal with cancer with a loving partner, but many of us take that journey on our own. Sadie has much to teach us about self-acceptance and creatively living life.

SADIE, AGE 71

I have had to confront bladder cancer in the past few years. Chemo didn't get rid of it, so I had major bladder and bowel surgery, which left me with lifelong side effects and daily pain. The surgery scars make my stomach look like the face of a Cabbage Patch Kid. The new look makes me apprehensive about being naked during intimacy. I am a pretty upfront person, and most likely, if a potential lover is put off by a part of me, then she doesn't get to enjoy the rest of me either.

Sexual feelings these days are rare, but they are still a vital part of me as I age. My sexual activity at the moment is with myself. I pleasure myself through touch, massage, masturbation, or sleeping outside in nature on a warm summer's night. The wonders in nature are filled with sexual energies. The osprey's swooping wings as it dives for a fish in the ocean, the warmth of a caterpillar on my arm—all of these wonders bring an excitement to my life.

Finding a woman who wants to enjoy her body and sexual pleasure as much as I do is the difficult part. It is still not the easiest thing for lesbians to find each other. A woman who is healthy about her sexuality and open enough to talk about it directly would be a prize to behold. It's not impossible; it just takes patience and openness. I wasted a lot of my life staying in relationships where I was not happy. Never again. A healthy relationship takes problem-solving, listening skills, courage, and the willingness to ask for what you want.

I have spent my life giving to others; now it's my turn to give to me. All I want now is to be calm about this part of my journey. I am not only taking baby steps—I feel like I am a fetus in the womb. I am hoping to be able to birth her with a new and energized view of living my life. I've got to love myself;

that's more important than trying to find someone to do that for me. It's exciting to feel energized about this reality, which has taken seventy-one years to learn and accept.

13

Erectile Dysfunction:
What Men Don't Say Out Loud

I KNOW MOST OF you men hate to go the doctor—and once there, you'd rather have your toenails extracted than talk about intimate concerns such as erectile function (or the lack thereof).

Talking with your partner can seem just as intimidating. But you must, men! You can have a fulfilling sex life with or without erections, but it takes honest and often repeated conversations with your doctor and your partner, as well as a new way of looking at sexual expression and satisfaction. Please let this chapter be your first step.

Nag, Nag, Nag: See Your Doc!

I know that admitting erectile difficulties to your physician might seem about as palatable as announcing it at your class reunion, but please tell your doctor. You may be taking a medication that interferes with erections (such as diuretics, antihistamines, blood-pressure medications, antidepressants, or cancer treatment). Erectile dysfunction (abbreviated as "ED") may also be caused by cardiovascular disease, diabetes, testosterone deficiency, prostate-cancer treatment, or diseases of the nervous system, such as multiple sclerosis or Parkinson's. Smoking decreases blood to the penis. Excessive alcohol consumption can cause nerve damage and erectile dysfunction too.

That's just the beginning of the list.

See why it's important to find out what's going on? Your doctor can tell by examining you and testing hormone levels what the cause might be, and what treatment is likely to get you back in the saddle. And wouldn't that be a good thing?

ADVICE FROM AN EXPERT
What's Causing Your ED?
BY LOREN A. OLSON, MD

Erectile difficulty happens occasionally to every man. A man who fails to have an erection more than 50 percent of the time would get the clinical diagnosis of erectile dysfunction.

Erectile problems occur for a variety of reasons—including stress, fatigue, alcohol, and conflict in relationships. It occurs more frequently with age, as testosterone declines. As we mature, sexual arousal is slower and generally requires greater stimulation. Recovery time between sexual encounters is longer. Distractions like painful joints lead to erectile failure more frequently. However, erectile failure should never be considered normal.

To determine if declining testosterone levels are a factor in erectile functioning, see your doctor for a physical exam, including a rectal prostate examination. You'll probably also get laboratory tests that include the following:

➤

➤

- testosterone level

- thyroid function

- luteinizing hormone (a pituitary hormone that tells the testes to produce more testosterone)

- PSA (prostate-specific antigen; for prostate cancer)

One of the major issues affecting sexual functioning is "performance anxiety." Men are socialized to believe that real men don't fail at sex. Once a man has struggled with achieving an erection, he often becomes preoccupied with a fear of failure. This fear begins to displace the focus on pleasure and further interferes with sexual functioning.

Once the concern "Will I be able to get it up?" enters the mind, the struggle usually accelerates. Some men try to increase the pace of the sexual encounter, out of fear that they might fail to maintain their erection—but that makes the problem escalate even further. Fear of failure often leads to avoidance of sex in a relationship.

REED, AGE 50

My erections are not as strong or hard as when I was younger. I now need direct physical stimulation to get an erection, instead of becoming erect while kissing or touching my wife. Once my penis is erect, I need steady, direct stroking—with my hand, or my partner's—to have an orgasm. When I try to have intercourse, I find the stimulation is not enough for me to reach orgasm. I lose my erection without direct touching of my penis. Also, I am visual: Seeing my penis being stroked and seeing myself ejaculate are very erotic to me.

Erectile Dysfunction Medication and Your Relationship

BY DAVID HERSH, MD

Only about half of men with erectile concerns seek treatment. Many doctors are as hesitant as their patients to bring up the question about erectile function.

If you are having any difficulty in achieving or maintaining an erection, I encourage you to see your physician. In addition to achieving an erection, it may save your life. Erectile-dysfunction issues may be a signal of serious disease, including clogged arteries or high blood pressure.

Three drugs on the market are effective for both physical and psychological causes of erectile problems. These drugs improve the erectile function of your penis, but you'll still require sexual stimulation to bring about a useful erection for intercourse. All the good old inputs are necessary: your partner, your mood, the setting, and other erotic stimuli.

Please proceed with caution, and examine where erectile-enhancement drugs fit into your relationship. Medication is not a complete cure for sexual problems. Erectile problems are best treated with both medication and sexual therapy.

Be completely open and honest with your physician and pharmacist, and please only take these drugs with a prescription by your physician. Do not buy them over the Internet or borrow them from your friend. Never combine different medications for the treatment of erection problems.

Some men do not initiate sex because they fear they will fail to get a firm erection. Greater confidence and erections

➤

mean a more satisfying sex life. But please don't just pop one pill, get a poor erection, and feel the medication and you have failed. You need to give the medication four or five tries to have a good idea whether it will help you. Anticipation, the anxiety of the situation, and performance expectations can make the first attempts less than perfect. Call your physician if you have any questions or problems.

Beware of unrealistic expectations. These drugs will enhance your erection, but they will not increase either your sexual desire (libido) or the receptivity of your partner. They will not make you desire your partner more, make you a better lover, or increase your passion. Medication cannot improve relationships or self-esteem. But a therapist can.

ED or EDis?

Sex educator Michael Castleman understands the sexual concerns of men: From 1991 to 1995, he answered the sex questions submitted to the *Playboy* Advisor. Here he explains the difference between erectile dysfunction (ED) and erection dissatisfaction (EDis).

ED and EDis

BY MICHAEL CASTLEMAN, MA

True erectile dysfunction (ED) is the inability to raise an erection, despite vigorous extended hand massage of the penis. Only a small fraction of men from the age of forty-five to sixty have true ED. A larger but still-modest fraction of men over sixty have true ED.

True ED is usually the result of a medical problem—either a problem with the nerves that control erection, or more likely, a narrowing of the arteries that carry blood into the penis. Like the arteries of the heart, the arteries into the penis can become narrowed by atherosclerotic plaques. Causes of plaque formation include the following: heart disease, diabetes, smoking, high blood pressure, high cholesterol, a high-fat diet, and a sedentary lifestyle. In other words, all risk factors for heart disease are also risk factors for ED. In addition, ED can be caused or aggravated by stress and anxiety, which constrict the arteries and limit blood flow into the penis.

While only a fraction of men over forty-five experience true ED, just about every man experiences what sex therapists call erection dissatisfaction (EDis). Men with EDis can still have erections, but they don't rise as quickly as they used to. They no longer rise from fantasy alone. Men begin to need direct penis stimulation by hand or mouth. When erections rise, they may not look or feel as firm as they were in your twenties. They may also droop from minor distractions—anything from donning a condom to hearing a motorcycle roar up the street.

➤

The good news is that EDis is a normal and natural part of aging. If older erections wilt a bit, hand massage and/or oral stimulation bring them back up again—if you remain relaxed and patient. If you get stressed and anxious, this reduces the likelihood of a return to a fuller erection.

Most older men are unclear on the distinction between true ED and EDis. Many mistakenly think they have ED when they experience the normal age-related erection changes of EDis.

EDis, however, can be disconcerting. I've been a sex educator for thirty years. I knew all about what happens to erections after fifty. Despite my knowledge, when those changes started happening to me, I found them unnerving.

Erection medication (Viagra, etc.) helps treat EDis. In fact, most men who take erection drugs don't have true ED. They have EDis.

Many men with female partners fear that they can't please her without an erection, or they give up on sex altogether. But the woman's pleasure organ is the clitoris. Many women prefer cunnilingus to intercourse. Women know that an erection and vaginal insertion are not necessary or sufficient for sexual pleasure and orgasm. But many men don't know this.

Men with erectile dysfunction or erectile dissatisfaction need to reframe their thinking about sex. I've spent my life as a sex educator and counselor trying to persuade men that they'll have better sex and get better response from women if they ditch their preoccupation with their penis and focus instead on leisurely, playful, whole-body, massage-based sensuality. If you're interested in staying on the path of self-discovery, seeing a sex therapist can really help.

DOCBOB, AGE 72

My ability to share intimacy with my wife is not limited to my penis! We play and joyfully follow, no matter where the path leads. Sex in later years should not be dependent on flawless intercourse. The broader concept of lifelong sexuality must include pleasure in sensual touch and loving communication. I have given up downhill skiing and probably will never white-water raft again. I have not given up on intercourse yet, but I have moved beyond it. When that ability goes, I will still savor the pleasure of a loving caress.

Talking about ED

Prostate-cancer survivor and healthcare educator Rabbi Ed Weinsberg and his wife gradually adapted to his ED through explicit discussions and lots of touching, kissing, and cuddling. They changed from a focus on intercourse—which had dominated through thirty-four years of marriage—to a more emotional and spiritual intimacy. Here he offers tips for talking to your doctor about medical possibilities, and about reframing how you think about sex with your partner.

ADVICE FROM AN EXPERT
Sex after ED
BY RABBI ED WEINSBERG, EDD, DD

Some 20 percent of American men—as many as thirty million—contend with erectile dysfunction. Many of these men also have a low libido: a severely diminished sex drive, preventing arousal.

Included in the group of men with ED, and often accompanied by a low libido, are the majority of the 2 million prostate cancer survivors in the United States alone. At least 80 percent were diagnosed with early-stage prostate cancer and treated through surgery or radiotherapy, as well as other medical techniques. Most of these men have benefited from erectile nerve-sparing. Many will be able to continue achieving erections and will be able to raise their libidos to some extent. It's crucial to talk openly with your urologist and other healthcare providers about your options.

Get guidance from your urologist to address your concerns. Address your sexual concerns with your urologist, before and after a health procedure. Four types of prescribed drugs or devices offer most men temporary relief from ED, and your doctor can explain which are appropriate for your condition:

- Viagra or other PDE-5 inhibitors

- VED (vacuum erection device, or "penile pump")

- Caverject (alprostadil) injections

- MUSE pellets

➤

Doctors can also explain how Kegel exercises can help men as well as women gain greater sexual stamina.

Ask your doctor about raising your libido through testosterone or herbal supplements. Some doctors, nurse practitioners, and physician assistants will initiate discussions about ED with their patients before or after treatment. However, unless prompted by their patients, relatively few urologists or their staff offer patients guidance for treating a low libido. Find out if you can safely raise your libido by taking a testosterone or herbal supplement in the appropriate prescribed amounts. Doctors usually do not prescribe testosterone for men until quarterly PSA testing demonstrates you are unlikely to get prostate cancer, or if periodic PSA screenings indicate you have been cured of cancer for at least two years following treatment.

Decide to "make love," rather than "have sex." Physical intimacy is possible and important to your relationship, whether or not you can have intercourse or orgasm. Orgasm is possible for most men, with or without an erection.

Your manhood does not depend on your capacity for intercourse. Instead make your main objective to bond together as a couple, physically and emotionally. It's understandable that losing sexual functioning as you've experienced it most of your life can lead to a sense of emasculation. Yet if you accept that "making love" rather than "having sex" is at the core of your most intimate moments, sexual satisfaction is indeed possible. This is a way to reframe what intimacy is all about. Being affectionate from day to day, in every way, is the best kind of foreplay.

The Benefits of Therapy

Although I can't emphasize enough the importance of seeing a doctor if you're having erectile difficulties, ED affects the emotions as well, and a therapist is also helpful.

KENNY, AGE 71

My wife passed away almost four years ago. We were married for forty-five years. After two years, I started dating seriously. I knew I had to get back out there.

The problem is that I cannot maintain an erection to enter a lady. I have learned to tell my partner up front that the plumbing may or may not work. It is disheartening to go flaccid at the point of penetration. I was recently told by a date that I have not let go of my wife yet. I think she is right.

My doctor and my urologist both diagnosed me with ED and prescribed Cialis. I take the pills, but it doesn't really solve my problem. I don't think that I have ED—I have no problem achieving or maintaining an erection except when I attempt insertion. I personally think it goes further than that. I suspect that I need some sort of therapy.

Joan Responds

Kenny, I'm glad you went to a doctor, but I'm not happy about what you learned—or, more accurately, what you didn't learn. ED isn't a final diagnosis—it's a symptom of an underlying problem. Did they run tests, make sure your heart is fine, and look at hormone levels?

You know you need counseling because your date's suggestion rings true to you. It makes sense to me that your grief is affecting your sexuality. Have you looked into starting therapy? You may be amazed at how helpful it is.

An Update on Kenny

I received this happy update from Kenny two and a half months later.

I have been seeing two therapists: a talk therapist and a hypno-therapist. The talk therapist made me realize that I was not grieving for my wife but for myself. Through discussions with her, I have changed my lifestyle around. I put away most of the pictures and reminders of my wife that I had all over the house. I started to redecorate my house with a more masculine decor.

The hypnotherapist took me back through my life and made me see events that occurred in my childhood that had shaped the person I became. Then I was able to put these past occurrences out of my mind and concentrate on now.

Since going to these therapists, I have had much more successful interactions with the women that I date. I can discuss freely what I feel and expect from a relationship. I am having a lot more fun, and I enjoy each day.

And I do not have the problem with ED that I once did. Penetration is not a problem anymore, and sex is much more enjoyable. I have to thank my therapists for that. They have brought me a long way in just two and a half months.

Please warn all your gentlemen about the dangers of ED medica-tion. It can cause temporary or even permanent blindness. I am suf-fering a cloudlike obstruction to my vision in the lower-left quarter of both eyes. The doctors say it will probably correct itself in time. This is caused by a drop in blood pressure, causing a neuropathy to the optic nerve. The doctors give out samples and prescribe these medications, but they do not always tell you about the side effects. The occurrences are rare, but they can happen.

Beware of Fake ED Meds

Never buy ED meds over the Internet. They may be fake, and they may be fatal. Yes, I'm trying to scare you, guys. Men who buy phony drugs for erectile dysfunction face significant risk from hazardous contents, according to an international review of the counterfeit drug industry, published in the January 2010 issue of *International Journal of Clinical Practice.*

An estimated 2.3 million ED drugs are sold monthly without a prescription, and 44 percent of online Viagra purchases are fake, this study reveals. Phony pills may include harmful ingredients such as amphetamine, commercial paint, bulk lactose, metronidazole, and even printer ink. Men who bought what they thought was Viagra or a herbal substitute have been found comatose or dead.

It's not worth saving a few dollars to risk death for a cheaper erection. And it's a very bad idea to bypass your physician and go straight to these drugs without a prescription, which should be given following a careful examination of your condition and your medical history.

Know This about Women, Men

Men tell me they don't believe it when their women partners say they can enjoy good, loving, exciting, and satisfying sex together even if the man doesn't get hard. Women tell me their male partners are so embarrassed and depressed about the lack of erections that they would rather give up on sex than be sensual and sexual together. Men: It isn't a hard penis that gives the women orgasms and contentment.

Men: As you discovered decades ago, women are different in how they like to be touched by fingers and tongue, and by what techniques or pace takes them over the top. If you ask, some women will tell you—straightforwardly or shyly—how to bring them to orgasm with your hand or your mouth. Others have difficulty expressing what they need, or they don't want you to feel inadequate by "instructing" you. Lou Paget offers some techniques that are almost certain to please. (Please also read the next chapter, where women talk about ED.)

ADVICE FROM AN EXPERT

Give Your Woman Fabulous Orgasms . . . Without an Erection

BY LOU PAGET

Gentlemen, most women actually orgasm most easily from manual and oral sex. Try these techniques.

Tips for Stimulating a Woman Manually

Slow is the name of the game. Women's sexual response cycle requires build, then plateau, then build again, then plateau. Too much sensation too quickly can result in crossing a razor-thin line into pain, and then the entire lovemaking session will be interrupted, if not ended.

Have clean hands, because the salt in normal sweat on your fingers may give her a burning sensation. Be sure your nails are smooth and short. (FYI: Before ever having sex with you, a woman will probably look at your hands, imagining them on her body. If she can't imagine them there, you may be out of luck and you won't know it's just a simple grooming issue.)

Use a good lubricant. The delicate genital tissues need to be kept moist. I suggest Very Private Intimate Moisture

➤

for postmenopausal women, as it closely matches their own natural lubrication.

Use a circular and back-and-forth motion with finger pads over the entire genital area to bring sensation into the genitals. (This may be your preferred prelude to oral.) Go into more clitoral-focused stroking after a minute, and then move back to the outer areas, then back in. Keep the cycles of "build, then plateau" in mind.

Assume this position, facing one another: either you are both seated, or you're seated and she's lying down, her legs outside yours, your genitals almost touching. Use the head of your nonerect penis to stroke up and over her clitoris. Apply lubricant as needed to both of you. The head of your penis has the firm/soft, warm texture that most women love.

Oral Play, Using the Tahitian (Kivin) Technique

Originally presented by Dr. Patti Britton in Paris, this is a take-it-home move. It will definitely enhance your oral repertoire.

1. Have her lie down and get comfortable. All she has to do is relax into the sensation. Align yourself at her hips at a right angle to her body. You will be on your stomach, resting on your elbows, your chin just above her genitals.

2. Use your upper hand to gently move the pubic hair area to expose her inner lips and clitoris.

3. Gently shift her legs open and raise her knee closest to you, so you can slip your bottom hand underneath and put your middle finger on her perineum (a.k.a. the "C point," the area below the entry into

the vagina, just above her anus). Do not move that finger—it is your feedback loop.

4. Your tongue motion will go straight across the clitoral hood, stroking the clitoral ridge from one side to the other. The intense stimulation comes from the tongue stroking across both arms of the clitoral nerves on either side of the clitoral glans. You may also feel two tiny raised dots on either side of the clitoral glans ridge, the "K points." Use those as your orientation spots for your tongue strokes, going back and forth between them over the clitoris. (Some women also require a form of penetration with a finger or a toy in order to orgasm. Varying oral strokes can be added, but keep the across-the-glans stroke going.)

5. When you feel the preorgasmic contractions at her C point, you'll know your tongue is stroking exactly the right place for maximum pleasure.

Chances are she will have a stronger and quicker orgasm than with the usual up-and-down strokes. The clitoris is actually ten to fifteen times bigger than the nub that you see, and stimulating both arms of the clitoral nerves leads to powerful orgasms.

The Most Important Sexual Statistic

BY MICHAEL CASTLEMAN, MA

Only 25 percent of women are consistently orgasmic during vaginal intercourse—no matter how long it lasts, no matter what size the man's penis, and no matter how the woman feels about the man or the relationship. This statistic comes not from just one study, but from a comprehensive analysis of thirty-three studies over the past eighty years by Elisabeth Lloyd in her fascinating book *The Case of the Female Orgasm* (Harvard University Press, 2005).

About half of women sometimes have orgasms during intercourse. About 20 percent seldom or never have orgasms during intercourse. And about 5 percent never have orgasms, period. In other words, intercourse is not the key to most women's sexual satisfaction.

Now, I'm not knocking intercourse. If it's well lubricated and men don't plunge in before women feel ready, it can be great fun. It makes many lovers feel deeply connected. But intercourse is not the essence of lovemaking.

Most women need direct clitoral stimulation to experience orgasm. They don't get it during intercourse, because the clitoris is located outside the vagina, under the top junction of the vaginal lips. Intercourse simply does not provide enough direct clitoral stimulation to arouse women enough to have orgasms. The key to erotic pleasure comes mostly from direct clitoral stimulation, using the fingers, palm, tongue, or sex toys. It's fine to have sex without intercourse, and many older couples decide they prefer it.

TOLDMAN, AGE 81

All men find their Joy Toy—their penis—early on. It took most of my lifetime to learn better ways of pleasuring a woman, and those ways weren't hanging between my thighs. Too bad that lots of men overlook their oral penis—the tongue. It never lets me down, nor her either. That's one penis that keeps me feeling like a man, with no pressure to perform.

I have lived with ED for so long that it has become an old friend to me. Not being able to maintain an erection until the completion of penile–vaginal intercourse is not the cat's meow. We have been spoon-fed that penis-into-the-hole concept of human sexuality. I used to feel lower than a snake's belly when my penis wouldn't stand up and be counted.

But an erection really is a moot point in giving women orgasms, and my oral penis can keep on licking and her orgasms will just keep on ticking. I do not have to depend upon an erection, and in pleasing her, I can have an unpressured orgasm all by myself.

I wish my partner knew that my genitals need a hell of a lot more manual pressure to bring me to arousal and to keep that arousal going. I would love to have a woman learn how I want her to play with my penis—to be a bit rough, as it isn't made off glass, and she won't break it. If women want an older man's penis to stay stiff, then they need to know that we need more vigorous pressure and hand-stroking.

Do I ask my partner for this? No. I am no better at telling her what I sexually want now than when I was a young buck. Why can't she just see that sex is giving and receiving?

BILL, AGE 70

I met a woman, and when attempting to have sex, I failed. No erection. Off to the doctor for a prescription. Viagra is not as advertised, at least for me. The pill gave me a nice erection, but it was like a piece of wood. No feeling, no climax, no going away. Later I discovered I could get an erection if the lady prompted me adequately—not every time, but when it occurred, it was much, much better. Now I may have an erection when needed, or I enjoy pleasing my partner without one. One thing I learned as an oldie is that making love and having sex can be so much better than simply jamming something into someone. If I have an erection, good. If not, then there are other things to do that will bring enjoyment.

Dating with Assistance

BillyBob read *Better Than I Ever Expected* and wrote to tell me how much it helped him. He wrote frequently over three years to comment on my blog and contribute his story by email. After coming out of an unsatisfying marriage, he started dating and had this embarrassing experience.

BILLYBOB, AGE 62

I started dating a lady who told me that she liked to masturbate maybe three times in a row and two or three times a day, so I knew she liked sex. We went for dinner, then she wanted to go back to my motel. I took a Viagra after we got back to the motel, hoping it worked fast! It did its normal thing and got me sexually aroused, but not 100 percent.

This was the most embarrassing time I have ever had, all because of a misconception some women have. Women who do not know about Viagra think if you take it, you just get ramrod hard, and that no further stimulation is required. That's just plain wrong. Men still need stimulation along with the Viagra. The drug is not a sack of cement installer.

I was not about to masturbate myself in order to get it hard. Not in the presence of a woman. So, as it turned out, she turned me off instead of on. What a bummer. I had looked forward to our meeting and the possibility of finally enjoying good sex with someone who enjoys it.

All a woman needs to know about the drug is that you do things normally, using stimulation together. So please tell your readers what my experience was.

Joan Responds

Viagra sometimes helps, but it doesn't increase libido or substitute for all those other crucial components of good sex that we all crave—touching, kissing, bonding, stimulating each other physically and emotionally, and enjoying each other's pleasure, as well as our own.

As embarrassing as this experience was for you, I'm sorry you didn't feel you could communicate your needs and desires to your partner. I hope she would have been happy to help you get aroused if she had understood. It's hard to understand why she didn't seem interested in stimulating you, just as part of the sex play (with or without Viagra), since that's a good part of the fun of sex.

The idea of masturbating in front of a woman to show her what you needed was too embarrassing for you. But as a woman, I find it very pleasurable and exciting to watch a man stimulate himself. I don't know if your partner would have reacted this way—I hope so, though.

It's always a good idea to communicate candidly with a new lover before sex actually gets going, and before popping the anticipatory Viagra.

DONALD, AGE 80

At sixty, I had performance anxiety with a twenty-years-younger companion, and it led to premature ejaculation. At seventy, I had the same anxiety with a ten-years-younger companion, and it led to the use of Viagra for ED. Now all is well! I don't think of myself as being old. Sex is still good at eighty! Blessings on Viagra. Don't be embarrassed to ask a doctor about using it.

RALPH, AGE 75

Two years ago, I got prostate cancer and went through a series of forty-two radiations. I "healed" my cancer but was left without the ability to achieve an erection. I still maintain the desire to be in a sexual, loving relationship.

I've had the problem look me in the face many times. Women say, "It doesn't matter." It sure as hell does. I have found that once I get that far into a relationship, my partner has expectations (which she is entitled to), and it better be there.

I've tried many solutions, with and without a partner. It is difficult to solve the problem alone, but you've got to do it, just in case you find a partner. No solution, no partner. The pills and supplements either gave me major side effects (dullness, blurry vision, or headaches) or simply did not work.

I personally have found that needle injections work for me. Problem solved? Not exactly. Here are the new problems: Injections are very expensive ($680 for twenty injections). They are age-dated and can expire, becoming noneffective. They have to be kept refrigerated. This can be a tough one when dating and not knowing the possibilities. Do you carry a needle and serum? If so, how and where do you carry it? How do you excuse yourself to get it and give yourself the injection?

Once you inject yourself, it takes twenty minutes of fore-play to become effective. And the reaction is not the same every time. Sometimes the recommended dosage does not always do the job, and you risk chance of failure again.

These problems leave me with great confusion and hesitation about even seeking a relationship. Dating is not about sex, but once dating is started, there are natural reactions that go with it. I inform the woman of my sexual limitations early in the relationship. This establishes an open communication and allows her to choose whether she wants to get involved. Also, it allows her to open up and disclose her own sexual limitations. Let's face it: A senior citizen is not a twenty-year-old anymore, and a lot changes in our bodies.

An understanding woman can help take the stress out of the situation. She can invite you to bring the injection into the house and refrigerate it. If there is going to be sex, she can suggest when it is time to get an injection. And if the injection doesn't work completely, her true understanding is very rewarding for the relationship.

I don't think many men are using injections to help their ED. When I tell other guys about the injections, they are usually ignorant of the subject and often reply, "Ouch."

CARL, AGE 86

I have erectile problems but I love my sex. I have a vacuum pump that works good. Nothing beats the good old lust. I have to have her lie on her back and get her legs up so I can insert my penis in properly. I can't use Viagra because I take nitro-glycerin. Maybe I am too old at eighty-six to carry on like this, but I love it.

Gay Men Talk about ED

I realize this chapter seems heterosexually oriented. I didn't plan it that way. Many more straight than gay men were willing to share their stories about ED, and many women sent me questions about their male partners. Thus the chapter evolved. Fortunately, Redhawk and Myron were generous about sharing their experiences as gay men.

REDHAWK, AGE 62

I don't get erections as easily as I once did, and they don't last as long. I have discovered many ways to enjoy being sexually alive with a flaccid dick. My whole body is an erogenous zone. I've learned to be patient with myself and my dick's responsiveness. I'm not in a rush—I savor every moment of sensual delight with another man. I know my partners are satisfied when they leave with big grins on their faces and/or when they have their orgasm and howl. When there is an emotional and intellectual connection with my partner, it's all the more satisfying.

MYRON, AGE 57

My greatest fear about aging and sexuality has come and gone. What can be more fearsome sexually for a man than to have no sexual potency whatsoever, including very little ability to experience an erection? But I am over it. I play more than ever, but not with a sword.

I am bisexual in thought and desire but more gay in action and history. I used to be very sexual and easily aroused. Now my arousal is more emotional or takes place as a delight in the imagination. It is less of a strictly physical nature.

I have an AIDS diagnosis. Two years ago, my former sexual prowess dimmed incredibly, the blazing fire within dissolving into quiet smoldering ash. Possibly because of the different

HIV and heart medicines I take (with their mixed bag of side effects); or possibly because of the effects of HIV on sexual energy or depression, I experience a much-lessened ability to achieve a natural engorgement of the male member.

As a predominantly gay man, I can translate this easily into becoming a "bottom"—assuming a passive role, sexually, as opposed to my former "top" role. I am versatile and creative by nature, but the joy of heated arousal and explosion of juices no longer shakes my body and soul. It is a quieter experience.

The inability to achieve obvious arousal has become a challenge. The process of fluffing up is depressing. I find it sad to keep hacking away at something that no longer takes place. I have overcome this by being very loving with my partner. I focus on kissing, touching, embracing, and giving pleasure, instead of focusing on my own ejaculation, which does not happen anymore without an almost military effort. I have tried my share of sex-enhancing medical drugs. Most of them make me physically ill and no longer do much any damn way.

I have been dating someone younger who understands my limitations and is remarkably patient with me. The glory of our sexuality is that we can make out for hours and find amazing pleasure in simple touch. We have fun playing with verbal fantasies. When it comes time for him to be satisfied, we both know well how to achieve this, and that's that. He would very much like me to have the same kind of experience that he enjoys but has come to accept and embrace that it ain't gonna happen. So why beat ourselves up about it?

Fools my age don't sweat the details as much, and don't get as disappointed or turned off as quickly when things don't go our way. We, at an older age, can actually be wiser, more understanding, more nurturing, calmer, more adaptable.

14

Erectile Dysfunction:
Women Speak Out

I F YOU HAVE a partner with erectile difficulties, please read the preceding chapter before reading this one: It's always good to understand what's going on for *him* first. Then read this chapter, where you'll learn about the experiences of other women who are in your position. You'll also get expert tips to help you maintain, salvage, or resurrect a sexual relationship that will delight both of you. Please don't just let your sex life wither—it's not good for you, him, or your couplehood.

Whatever you do, don't just chalk it up to "old age" or pressure him to buy Viagra. The first step should be a medical exam and diagnosis. (See Chapter 13 for possible causes of erectile dysfunction.) I know that many men hate to see their physician for anything short of a severed leg, and admitting that he can't get it up might seem impossible, but do whatever it takes to get him to his doctor.

If your partner's ED has no physical cause, it might be due to an emotional issue, such as stress, performance anxiety, relationship issues, or trauma. Encourage him to seek counseling. It's never too late to learn, to grow, to overcome problems that seemed insurmountable, especially with you, his loving partner, at his side.

When He Won't Talk about It

I wish men felt comfortable about confiding in their partners, letting us support them emotionally and working with us to find creative solutions to erectile difficulties. But darn it, many don't. This section offers insight on why it's so hard for men to talk about erectile dysfunction, as well as solid advice on how to encourage them to open up about it.

ADVICE FROM AN EXPERT

What Men Feel—but Don't Say—about ED

BY MICHAEL CASTLEMAN, MA

Few women really understand how men feel when erectile difficulties develop. A part of his body he took for granted doesn't work like it used to. And this isn't just any part of the body. It's the body part that, in a profound way, defines him as a man.

Men have lived their whole lives taking their penises for granted: See a sexy woman, get hard. See porn, get hard. Think a sexual thought, get hard. Then all of a sudden, they're in a situation where they expect to have to rearrange their underwear to accommodate some swelling down there, and then . . . nothing happens.

Many men don't understand what's happening to them or why. But even those who do—me for example—feel surprised,

➤

upset, disappointed, depressed. When changes concern the penis, men get seriously freaked out.

It takes most young men years—decades—to leave penis-centric sex behind and understand the erotic value and pleasure of whole-body sensuality, rather than just sticking it in somewhere. Men who continue to view sex as penis-centered often think it's the end of sex when their penis stops behaving as they expect.

In my experience as a sex counselor and writer, I've found that few women appreciate how diminished men feel by ED. Men feel things just as deeply as women. Men are socialized to be the "strong silent type," to deny what they're feeling and just go on. Men get less practice than women discussing their emotions, and when they do, they're less skilled.

When the erections they took for granted their entire lives start to fail them, they freak. It's almost unthinkable. Some fear that their partners will view them as less than real men. So why talk about it? Why invite her to rub his nose in the fact that he's less of a man?

KATE, AGE 58

How can my husband and I get our sex life back? It used to be fantastic—several times a week. We were so much in love, and so willing to please each other. I told him that sex was one of the best parts of our relationship, and I never wanted us to lose the intimacy.

Then, around the time of our fourth wedding anniversary, he began having erectile problems, and the sex just stopped. I have been honest with him by saying I miss this aspect of our relationship, and asking him why he doesn't feel the same. But he absolutely refuses to discuss it. Every time I bring up the subject, he finds a way to change it. I'm afraid if we don't do something soon, we will just give up and lose our sex drives altogether.

Our relationship is wonderful in every other way. He is affectionate: He holds my hand, tells me he loves me, kisses me—although not passionately. However, I truly miss the special closeness we shared when making love. And although my libido has somewhat waned lately, I still have urges.

I love him madly and don't ever want to hurt him. It's just so hard to lose the intimacy I thought we'd always have. I feel my sex organs drying up and withering away. Any suggestions for how I can get our love life back on track?

Experts Respond

LIBBY BENNETT, PSYD, AND GINGER HOLCZER, PSYD

It's great that you have so much love for each other, and that you're both still affectionate with one another. The first order of business needs to include a physical exam for your husband, if he hasn't already done this. Erectile issues can be treated, but they may also be indicators of physical problems. Perhaps the physician might encourage your husband to try an erection aid, like Viagra. Coming from a doctor, this advice may be more easily accepted by your husband as an appropriate intervention. Keep in mind, however: Your husband can have an orgasm even without an erection.

Open the lines of communication using "we" instead of "you" in expressing your concerns: "How can we become a more satisfied and connected couple? I want us to look for solutions together."

Express your need to continue discussing this issue so that you don't begin to resent his silence. You might say, "I know we've talked about our sexual issues before, and it seems frustrating to you. Would you be willing to sit with me today and talk a moment? I want you to know that I still need to explore this issue with you."

We encourage you to read about sensate focus exercises. These are designed to help couples reconnect with one another, without the focus of performance, erections, or orgasms. A typical sensate focus exercise would include sensual massage with various textures and techniques, such as feathers, lotions, ice cubes, fabrics, rubbing bodies together, oral, or manual stimulation. Talk with your husband about using sensate focus to enjoy touch and playfulness without pressure to perform, reach erection, or achieve orgasm.

Express your appreciation to your husband for the continued affection and love that you feel. Surprise your husband with a date that might include an activity that you haven't done in a while. Go to the park. Picnic together. Make out in the back seat. Flirt with each other. Touch his leg under the table. Wear something sexy. Keep the flames burning.

MOLLY, AGE 63

I was in a long-term relationship that was wonderful—until he started to experience ED. His whole thinking and attitude changed. He thought if he couldn't get an erection, why bother? He completely cut me out of his life, wouldn't communicate with me in any way. I tried everything to get him to talk to me. I wish I could try to turn back time and make him understand that an erection is not everything in a loving sex life. I still love the man and I think I always will. It's so sad.

An Expert Responds

MICHAEL CASTLEMAN, MA

Around age fifty, most men's erections start to become iffy. And arousal—once instant and almost automatic—a woman smiles, he's turned on—becomes work. Either of these issues would be enough to push some men to "retire" from sex. But experiencing both erection and arousal difficulties together is very disconcerting and makes quite a few men figure that sex is over for them.

What's actually over is young sex. But older sex is still available if men are willing to make some adjustments—notably, learning how to enjoy sex with iffy erections or no erections, and taking much more time for eroticized play before getting into bed for sex.

These changes are a challenge for many men. I'm reasonably confident that a brief course of sex therapy—say, a dozen weekly sessions—could help you both come to a mutual accommodation about sex. To find a sex therapist near you, visit the American Association of Sex Educators, Counselors, and Therapists (www.aasect.org) or the Society for Sex Therapy and Research (http://sstarnet.org).

If it's difficult to talk about this, write him a letter expressing how you feel and offering your suggestion to go as a couple to sex therapy. If he won't go, then go by yourself. Going solo is suboptimal, but in many cases the therapist can help you deal with your own feelings and can make suggestions that might eventually persuade him to join you.

Facing Cancer and ED

Ever since my husband had his prostate removed because of prostate cancer, he has been reluctant to touch me. This is so upsetting. I love him very much and don't know what to do.

This is more common than you might realize. When a man discovers he can't have erections any more, especially when he's dealing with cancer, he sometimes turns his face to the wall and stops bonding or even talking. Cancer and sexuality specialist Anne Katz has these suggestions. (Please also see Chapter 12 for much more about sex and cancer.)

ADVICE FROM AN EXPERT

Starting the Conversation

BY ANNE KATZ, RN, PHD

Many men are deeply distressed by their inability to have an erection, and they may avoid all physical contact with their partner so as not to "lead them on" or disappoint them. This leads to a very unhappy partner who wants to express his/her love and support but feels cut off and cut out.

What is important is for the couple to *talk*. It is often difficult to talk about a sensitive topic when emotions are running high. But talking goes a long way to healing and connecting. Start with an "I" statement like "I miss touching you and being touched by you. How can we reconnect again?"

While there are medications and treatments that may help, further treatment should be a couple's decision. The man should always include his partner in medical appointments so that both people can express themselves and have their

➤

questions answered. Because communication is so important, the couple may need professional help to start the communication flowing. But seeking help is the first step.

Getting Past the Hurdles

Many of my readers have found ways to communicate and work around erectile difficulties. Read on to hear some of their success stories.

ASHLEY, AGE 75

My husband is eighty-eight. At his age, I'm happy that our sex life is active at all! We have intercourse and/or extended sex play once or twice a month, and affection and cuddling all the time. We have lots of sensual experiences that are not genitally focused. We give each other massages in front of the fireplace, we sleep naked, we take baths together together. We hold hands, cuddle, hug, and kiss.

My husband's physical changes have changed the nature and frequency of sex between us. He has taken Viagra and Cialis and has also injected Trimix into his penis to help him achieve a firm erection. But despite all of this, the erection does not last long, and sometimes all these ministrations don't work at all, which causes him great distress. Sex has always been important to both of us, and this is a disappointment for us both. I really appreciate his willingness to speak to his urologist about his sexual frustrations and to take the steps that he does.

He likes to please me, and fortunately, he has a nimble tongue and fingers. I find that if I get to a certain high level of arousal during sex with my husband and then masturbate, I can achieve a fully satisfying orgasm. It's like mountain-climbing—he helps me climb up almost to the mountaintop, but I need to summit on my own.

I know he is disappointed when he doesn't come himself. He sometimes says, "I guess sex is over for me." But then at other times—especially if we have not had sex for maybe a month—he does achieve orgasm and is happy again.

MARTHA, AGE 65

I've had men occasionally who couldn't get it up at first. It never worried me. Almost 100 percent of the time, a little oral stimulation got it right back up there—even with men who've told me they had trouble all the time with other women. Just knowing that it didn't bother me and that I was willing to work on it usually took care of it. My husband, when we first got together, would lose his hard-on just before penetration. I told him it was okay, that I was willing to take as much time as he needed. And guess what? He got a raging hard-on that lasted just as long as I needed it to, and we rarely had a problem after that!

Making Love without an Erection

With knowledge, understanding, and creativity, sex without an erection can be satisfying for both of you, and strongly bonding. This section features some snippets from women about the pleasures of making love, no erection required, as well as some excellent hands-on advice on how to expertly stimulate your man, whether or not he gets an erection.

CHARLENE, AGE 52

I took up dating with a passion and began having some great sexual relationships. I learned that ED in older men is not a handicap to joyful, passionate fun. I revived my youthful love of making out for long sessions and discovered that men love it too. They get gaga over great kissing. Many of them have been deprived for so long. One man said it was a revelation to be with someone who made him feel so lusty and passionate, erection or not.

TORY, AGE 65

One of my most wonderful relationships was with a man who was losing his sexual potency because of diabetes. He could get half an erection at best. He revealed this toward the beginning of our prerelationship correspondence. When we finally met, we had great sexual pleasure, and his potency improved over the month we spent together. He was never able to have a full erection, but he was always able to have orgasms, and this gave me great pleasure.

Sensual Sexplay: Massaging Your Man

BY SUSANA MAYER, PHD

Try this sensual massage on your male partner for his pleasure—and yours.

1. Focus on pleasuring his entire body. Many places on the body are erogenous zones, not just the genitals.

2. Use your fingertips, lips, or a cosmetics brush to find sensitive areas of your partner's body. Go slowly—sensually. You are looking for new spots to stimulate and excite.

3. Ask for verbal feedback—words or sounds—to help you know what parts of his body turn him on or off.

4. Once you have discovered the pleasure spots on his body, front and back, focus on stimulating one of these sensitive areas.

5. If your partner is still focused on his penis, massage this area and include stomach, thighs, testicles (most gently, please!), and anus.

6. Tell your partner that the goal isn't erection—that you would in fact prefer he remain soft for this massage, and that you truly enjoy him this way. He can take pleasure in the sensations of having his penis massaged without any goals. He might even orgasm in the process. (Men do not need a hard penis to orgasm.)

➤

7. Ask him not to touch you intentionally during the massage—it will interfere with the sensations he is receiving by dividing his focus.

8. You'll discover that you receive pleasure from being the creator of these wonderful sensations and observing his responses. It may arouse you too.

9. He can use the same techniques on you at another time.

Look wider than just your genitals for sexual pleasure—there is more pleasure for both of you to discover during sensual playtime.

MIRIAM, AGE 57

I don't need my partner to have an erect penis for me to have a great time. I need him to attend to my sexual pleasure, which can be accomplished even better with his fingers. I don't say this just to make him feel better. It's absolutely true. But I think men assume I'm just being kind, which ruins the relief they could feel if they truly accepted that I mean it. We'd both have a better time together in bed if they believed me.

Even without an erection, I enjoy:

- hours of carefree touching

- "let your fingers do the walking," which leads to wonderful orgasms

- kisses that touch the bottom of my soul

- gazing into each other's eyes

- sharing my arousal with him, and seeing him respond with the subtlest shift in his eyes as he appreciates what's happening for me—bliss.

Because I enjoy all of this even without my lover's erection, it is important to me that he teach me what he particularly finds pleasurable, sensual, and satisfying so I can attend to him. It wouldn't be as much fun if he only focused on me and didn't receive as well.

ROSEMARY, AGE 57

I love him no matter how he performs. He is a loving, giving man, and if he has difficulties with erections, it makes no big difference to me. I just want him to be happy. And he knows how to make me happy even if he does not have an erection— by manual stimulation and the use of a vibrator.

BREENA, AGE 59

My lover has some erectile difficulties and sometimes uses Levitra. I learned that how hard he was didn't accurately measure how turned on he was. I could tell that he really was turned on, and it was just his body not responding. The connection between us is what is important, so we just find what works for us.

Pleasuring Your Man When
He Doesn't Get Hard

BY LOU PAGET

In older age, a man's erection is not necessarily a direct indicator of his sexual interest in his partner. He may not get hard for a number of reasons that have nothing to do with your desirability or technique. The good news is that many men can experience "softgasms," orgasms without an erection.

Here are some oral and manual techniques that your partner will love, even if he can't show you with an erection. Above all, enjoy pleasuring your man. The more you're into it, the more he will be.

Manual Techniques

Just about any manual technique that worked for erect penises will work on softer penises with these adaptations.

- Choose a good lubricant. A silicone-based lubricant won't dry out like water-based lubes. The easier the flow of manual play, the more confident and connected you'll feel.

- Use his visual nature to your advantage. Prop him up with pillows, so he can watch you play with him. Generously apply lubricant to both hands, and then imagine you are rolling a thick bread stick as you apply the lubricant to him.

- Use firmer stimulation. Ask him to put his hand around yours and show you his preferred strength

➤

of hold. Once he is lubed, use one hand for an up-and-down stroking motion on the penis, and use your other hand at the base of the shaft to keep the penis at attention. You won't always need to go to the base of the shaft, and in general, it's better to keep the stroking rotation of your hands closer to the head, as the most sensitive area for most men is the frenulum (that quarter-sized V area on the underside of the head).

- Stroke up, not down. Many men masturbate using a firm stroke up the shaft—away from the base—as a way to get themselves hard. So use the firmer part of your stroking for the up-the-shaft stroke, not the descending stroke.

For a variety of manual moves, my book, *How to Be a Great Lover*, offers twenty-one different manual techniques, illustrated and described step-by-step.

Oral Techniques

Your hands and mouth are creating, in essence, an imposter vagina, but with more sensation, due to the pressure of your hands. Your mouth supplies the heat and the moisture. A technique sure to please is creating a hand tower, with your two hands stacked and then attached to your mouth. You now have an oral tube. Open your fingers and wrap them around his shaft. Use a gentle or firm suction in, and start an up-and-down-the-shaft motion while rotating your hands.

15

No Way Back:
When Your Partner Has
Alzheimer's Disease

M OST OF THE seniors I interviewed for this book are hoping
to improve the setbacks that are making their sex lives
and relationships less than ideal. One group, though, is unique,
because they hold no hope of reversing the condition that makes
their relationship sad and sexless: their partner's Alzheimer's
disease.

Alzheimer's disease and other types of dementia cause gradual
impairment in memory, thinking, language, and self-care skills.
The impaired partner can no longer reason, understand, communicate, or remember as he or she used to. A whole relationship
history may be slowly wiped out as the brain disease worsens
over a period of many years.

Books, support groups, and websites help the caregiving partner understand the disease and cope with caregiving responsibilities, with advice that always includes "get support for your
feelings" and "take care of yourself too."

But what about sex? Is it still possible when one partner has
Alzheimer's? Is it even desirable? And why is information about
this so sparse, even on the all-knowing Internet?

I wonder if caregiving partners even ask the doctor about sex. Or are they supposed to accept that their sex lives are over, along with the relationship as they once knew it? Do they feel shame at even thinking about sex as they watch their partner slip away? Do they go off quietly and masturbate in private—if they're not too tired from caregiving to even think about their own sexual needs? Do they take a lover?

My gratitude goes out to the spouses of loved ones with Alzheimer's who were willing to share their stories, and to Daniel Kuhn, MSW, former Director of the Professional Training Institute for the Alzheimer's Association–Greater Illinois Chapter, who served as consultant for this chapter.

For more information about Alzheimer's disease and other types of dementia, visit the Alzheimer's Association website, www.alz.org, or phone the 24/7 helpline: (800) 272-3900.

Changes in Sexual Relations with Alzheimer's Disease

Changes in sexual behavior are symptoms of the disease, not the person's character, the Alzheimer's Association (www.alz.org/national/documents/topicsheet_sexuality.pdf) points out. Some people may act out sexually; others may show no interest in sex whatsoever. Libido-reducing side effects of medications may also play a part. Both the impaired partner and the caregiving partner may experience depression—a sexual downer. Whether you feel sexy toward your partner or not, touching can still be nurturing and satisfying to both of you, and can give you a sense of intimacy.

How Does Alzheimer's Disease Affect Sexuality?

DANIEL KUHN, MSW

Sexuality is highly complex, and so are relationships. How you, as a couple, face the ongoing dilemmas posed by Alzheimer's disease can vary widely. You're likely to encounter one or more of these changes in your partner and in your own response to the relationship:

- The person with Alzheimer's disease may retain sexual desire and function for a period of time. You may still find sex to be satisfying, or you may be turned off by the many changes occurring in the relationship. You may be upset by your partner's chronic forgetfulness, repetitive questions, and growing dependency. You may be willing to participate in sexual activity in an effort to recapture part of the past relationship. Or you may resist sexual overtures, and your partner may feel rejected or diminished.

- The person with Alzheimer's may still have sexual desire but may be losing sexual function. You may be willing to help your partner engage in sexual activity. However, you may feel unsatisfied by acting as a coach or by extending the caregiving role to sexual activity.

- The person with Alzheimer's disease gradually loses sexual desire and functional capacity. You may wish to continue having sexual relations, or you may accept the changes in the impaired partner and let go of

➤

sexual relations. The fact that your partner is no longer willing or able to enjoy sex may prove unsatisfying to you.

- Rarely, the person with Alzheimer's disease exhibits hypersexuality, an incessant need to engage in sexual talk and activity. This problem poses major challenges and usually requires medical intervention to be resolved.

If your partner no longer initiates sex or is unresponsive to your sexual overtures, then the sexual part of relationship may no longer be satisfying for one or both of you. You will experience changes yourself as you cope with your partner's illness and your caregiving responsibilities. At any point in the disease process, you may find you no longer feel sexually attracted to your partner because of the many changes in the person and relationship.

How long you can or wish to maintain sexual relations will depend upon many things, particularly your ability to cope with the other changes in the relationship. Your partner may eventually become so cognitively impaired that shared intimacy, including sex, is problematic. At this point, focusing on nonsexual forms of intimacy may be more fulfilling and comforting for you and your partner.

When your partner reaches the advanced stages of the disease, he or she may no longer remember your name or the nature of your relationship. Consent to participate in sex may be no longer possible at this time. Experimenting with nonsexual forms of intimacy and finding new ways to connect nonsexually may be emotionally satisfying.

MARGARET, AGE 74

My sex life is alive only in my dreams. My husband, age eighty-seven, is in the advancing stages of dementia. I grieve the loss of sex and the loss of the man I love to Alzheimer's disease.

My husband still is a handsome man, but I wouldn't want to have sex with him now, even if he were able. It just doesn't seem right, being his caregiver. I have had a terrible struggle making sense of my caregiving of him, and I have trouble keeping a connection with him. He looks good, and we are still able to go out socially, take walks, go to the movies, visit with friends. It stops here.

At times, I mourn the end of my sexual life. At times, I am resentful. And yet I look at the man and feel a quick start of my heart as I see the essence of who he is and was. I feel pangs that this part of our life is really over. He shows affection by massaging my sore shoulder muscles when we settle down for the night. It is sometimes comfortable falling asleep by his side. I do feel a tremendous sexual feeling in the dream world at times.

The last four years of my life have been a slow, painful, frustrating passage into understanding, education, caregiving, and learning how to take care of myself. I have a lot of support through friends, the Alzheimer's Caregiver Support Group, and private counseling. But in some ways, I am completely alone. I go through the motions of responding to constantly repeated questions. I'm continually on alert to make sure he is safe, and I wonder what is next. When the lights go out at night, I lie in bed next to my husband and wonder who I am, what I am doing here, where is this going. I am frightened. Am I losing myself?

The Next Step

We're not dancing a waltz.
We take two steps forward, then two backward,
side step, break, and walk two steps.
We listen to the tune.
His fingers tap on his knee to the beat of the music
on the "oldies" radio station.
He plays a few notes on his stand-up bass.
Just this morning, he didn't have the name for a rose.
"Three of them in a vase."
Or, "The little cups down at the bank."
His writing, he thinks, is buried at his son's home.
Surreal.
Meaning disappears.
Fear appears.
The music plays.
"Break," he says when we're on the dance floor,
"Now, take two steps."
We come back together.
He has a firm grip on my waist. His hand
slides up my back.
He taps to the rhythm as if he were
Playing his stand-up bass.
He loves his music.
We wait for the next step.
    —Margaret

FRANCES, AGE 69

Do you believe in love at first sight? I do, because that is what happened with me and Orson. Over sixty, he had gray hair to his shoulders, funny black-rimmed half glasses perched on his nose, ratty blue jeans, and his bare toes stuck out of the oldest

Berkies I have ever seen. The glance from those brown eyes was like an electric shock.

Our first night together, he opened his arms to me and said for me not to be afraid, we belonged together. We were crazy in love with each other from the first moment, and were still in love at the last, twenty years later.

Our sex life was passionate—several times a day at first. Gradually, it became once a day and then maybe every other night. We both like to caress, hug, and kiss, and we rarely walked past each other without a touch or a pat. Usually on a lazy Sunday afternoon, he would massage me, ending with sex.

Orson was diagnosed with early Alzheimer's eight-and-a-half years before he died. We lost our business due to Orson's illness. Stress took its toll on our sex life. It's hard to feel sexy when you are wondering where you are going when your home is foreclosed. I began to carry these burdens of working, caring for him, and solving our legal problems. Sex was reduced to once a week, with very little foreplay or invention. My body was also changing, and I was dealing with extreme dryness by using vaginal creams.

When Orson was eighty—his Alzheimer's progressing—his internist wrote him a prescription for the little blue wonder pill. One night Orson had a prolonged erection which lasted for some time. I was under him while he was in a near frenzy. When I finally could get him off, I was badly torn and bleeding.

As Orson returned to his normal state and realized the extent of my injuries, he became distraught and started crying. I got out of bed, filled myself with vaginal cream, put on a pad, and changed the bloody bed. The following day, I went into my doctor. Orson went into a depression and wanted to kill himself. He threw the Viagra down the toilet. We both discussed the incident with his doctor, as well as talking privately with each other. He never wanted to have sex again.

I tried many times to talk about what happened with him, but he continued to blame himself for losing control. We went on hugging, kissing, and holding each other, but we never enjoyed intercourse or attempted any other type of sexual activity.

There came a time when it was necessary for Orson to go into extended care. The little old ladies loved him and he was usually surrounded by two or three. Once when I went to see him, he was holding the hand of a frail little woman and gently talking to her. The aide rushed over and wheeled him away. I wheeled him back and sat and talked to both of them. I saw no harm in him holding hands or socially touching another patient. It is a basic human need to be touched and shown affection.

I watched Orson die for over eight years. I grieved for him every night, and I still do. I was blessed with Orson's love. It really was for richer or poorer, and in sickness and health. I loved him then, and I love him now.

An Expert Responds

DANIEL KUHN, MSW

Prolonged erection, or priapism, is a well-known side effect of Viagra. Lesser-known side effects are the transient global amnesia and aggressive behavior that your husband also exhibited. When he returned to his "normal state," he was shocked that he had lost control over his behavior and harmed his wife.

Sadly, many people with Alzheimer's disease feel as if they are losing control over their lives, as memory, thinking, and language abilities become more impaired over time. This unfortunate incident perhaps only heightened Orson's fear of losing control over his life and may have further diminished his self-esteem.

For other readers in this situation: Depression should be treated aggressively, and sexual activity should not be initiated again unless the partner with Alzheimer's shows interest. The caregiving partner should also seek help in coping with the many changes in their marriage, as he or she needs and deserves support during this incredibly challenging time.

Going Outside the Marriage

Alzheimer's disease can progress slowly, and your partner may live for years in your care. You have to figure out how to take care of yourself too, and this includes sexually. Whether or not you take a lover outside of your marriage will depend on your personal values and needs, your marriage history, and—if this ever came up in your marriage—your understanding of what your partner would have wanted for you.

At a certain point, it's your decision, and whatever you decide is right. The Alzheimer's Association encourages you to "do what feels best for you," to not feel guilty about not being attracted to your partner because of his or her changes and the changes in your role, and to even "consider dating, if it feels right for you."

WILLIAM, AGE 71

I'm a fulltime caregiver for my wife of thirty-seven years, who has Alzheimer's. I watch as her brilliant, adventurous, loving soul slides, year by year, toward extinction. I don't know from day to day if I'm wise, patient, or strong enough for such a sad, helpless job.

For eight years I've also been in relationship with someone who is the love of my life. Her challenges, though different, are as difficult as my own. In the midst of intense stress, my lover and I provide each other safe haven. We celebrate ourselves and our erotic life.

Changes began for my wife in her late forties. At first they were minor and diffuse, merely confusing. We began to get nervous about her distractibility and puzzled by her repetitive storytelling. Over several years, our relationship changed. By about ten years ago, sex had ceased to be a part of our shared life. I was bewildered and in mourning. Something was profoundly wrong, but we were still four years from diagnosis.

One day, while I was away at a weekend workshop, my new love walked into the room, walked toward me, and we kissed. We were launched as simply as that. We had an afternoon of necking and a night of joining, all of it feeling predestined. Sometime in the hours between late afternoon and waking, tangled in our sleeping bags in the morning, we became a committed couple.

I went home and told my wife everything. We had always had a modestly open relationship. My new lover and I both pledged my wife absolute veto: If she became uncomfortable with our sexual connection, we'd end it.

Today, eight years later, I have never been closer to my wife. Our love, as her illness deepens, has never been stronger. It's not sexual—we seem like brother and sister—but the commitment is absolute.

And my partner and I have discovered ways to endure our stressful lives, and my health problems and hers—while remaining playful and impassioned. Our love is profound, our lovemaking ecstatic. My partner has been a lifesaver for my wife and me—contributing her skills to help us through a major, Alzheimer's-generated financial crisis—while I have helped her with some of her difficult challenges. We three are unexpectedly fortunate having one another.

Honesty, full disclosure, and compassionate love have served us well. Do I recommend to you something as untraditional as what we've done? No, it's far too individual for that. But I'd love to see the silences around life choices lifted. I'd love to see everyone be free to choose, to risk, to expand the social strictures on love, and on life.

Keeping the Love

After I lost Robert, people reached out to me—among them, blog readers whom I had never met. One of them, Jean Pulcini, wrote me this email two months after Robert died, telling me how her love for her husband, who had Alzheimer's, is still as strong as ever. Jean attached a lovely tribute she wrote for her husband and gave me permission to publish it here.

I read your story with a sense of bittersweet. How blessed you were to have known such love, and how sad to have lost it. Three years ago today, I buried my beloved husband of nearly fifty years. I was his caregiver for several years, because Alzheimer's took his mind from us long before God took his body. I believe I love him even more today than through all of those years. I now have time to think back over all of life's joys and sadness, which we shared as one. I remember events that were long ago tucked away in my heart. I dream the most marvelous dreams that put him once again in my arms. I do know the loss and pain you feel. We never really have enough time, do we?

"It's Another Beautiful Day," by Jean Pulcini

This is my humble attempt to understand what is going on in the world of my husband of forty-seven years. My love has Alzheimer's. This disease has taken the heart and soul of a man and left a shell.

In the beginning I found myself denying the obvious—something is not quite right, is it? Little by little, the "not quite right" becomes a pattern, and that pattern grows each day. My anger, resentment, and frustration soon followed clinical diagnosis. I have come to terms with my emerging feelings. I, the caregiver, must remain sane. My time is no longer my own. The life I shared with my husband is now a memory only to me.

My husband was always a kind and gentle man, and he remains so. He takes direction without complaint and gives abundant thanks. He tells me of his undying love and compliments me. Actually he is more open about his feelings in that area than before the illness set in. He is constantly saying he is sorry for any mistakes he might make.

I know that he must be very confused, and he stays by my side to feel secure. Perhaps I also need him by my side to feel secure—letting go isn't an easy process, especially when the physical being is present and the mental being has long since abandoned its body. I yearn for the past and for a future.

It is my desire that my husband stay here in our home as long as it is possible. The lake, garden, and birds make up most of our world today. When we are able to be with family and friends, the sun shines a little brighter. As for now, in the words spoken by my husband every morning, "It's another beautiful day!"

VERONICA, AGE 72

About forty years into our marriage, Robbie was diagnosed with Alzheimer's disease. I discovered a well of strength in me that I had no idea existed. The last two years were absolutely dreadful, but I never broke down or hinted that I could not go on. I've been blessed with the gift of faith, so I knew where that well of strength was coming from. I dealt with every crisis with patience and love and fortitude.

The surprise was how much I loved Robbie. You don't realize how much you love someone until you are required to do things for them that you never in your life dreamed you would do. Even when your body is totally exhausted from 24/7 caregiving, you draw on your emotional and spiritual wells to discover that your love is still strong and enduring. It's like a special little gift given just to caregivers.

My advice for others whose partners have Alzheimer's? Make every effort to stay in the moment. Try not to dwell on how things used to be. Look at your loved one with the same love that you had when you fell in love. Because the disease turns them into a stranger, this is easier said than done. Find ways to nurture yourself, and find joy in your own life.

Robbie died three years ago, and as hard as the last years were, losing him was almost more than I could bear. This past year, I finally started to feel it's okay to laugh again, to go out and have fun. I discovered line dancing! Life has become a joy again, each new day an adventure and a gift. As I approach the fourth anniversary of Robbie's death, I know that his love will live in my heart forever. And now it's Veronica's time to pursue her dreams.

16

Death, Grieving . . . and Then What?

D URING MY EXTREME grief after Robert died, I cried all day. That's an understatement: I wailed, I screamed, I keened. I exploded in great, ripping waves of crying that felt like I was vomiting tears uncontrollably from my gut. My heart was being sawed to pieces. Those of you who have experienced the loss of your great love know what I'm talking about.

My sharp heart pain actually landed me in the emergency room one day. After test after test showed no physical problem, the doctor sat by my bedside and took my hand. "Has anything happened in your life recently?" he asked.

"Yes. My husband died."

"What does that feel like?"

"Like my heart is breaking," I sobbed.

Getting Help from a Grief Counselor

I didn't go to *a* counselor—over the first fifteen months, I had multiple sessions with two therapists, two grief specialists, and three support groups. At different times of my grieving, different opportunities were available to me via hospice, my HMO, and community resources. If your grief is dire, please don't white-knuckle it without help. These folks know what we're going through. They know how to listen to our pain and guide us to our next step of healing. This is their day job, and they do it really well.

Interestingly, my hospice grief counselor turned out to be someone I had dated a couple of times about twelve years earlier. At our first appointment, he looked into my eyes and said, "I remember how your smile used to light up your face. You'll get that light back."

My healing was accelerated by a daylong workshop held by Joe Hanson, a grief coach. One of his exercises transformed my thinking. He asked us to write the story we were telling ourselves about our loss, in one sentence. Then he helped us rewrite (he called it "reframe") the story so that it served us better going forward. Here's what I mean:

My original story: "I lost the love of my life, and my life is and will be empty without him."

My reframed story: "I found the love of my life and learned how to experience love fully, and I take this with me on my path."

See the difference? It's not just semantics—it's a whole different way of facing life from here on. Here's how Joe Hanson explains it.

Reframing Our Grief Story

BY JOE HANSON

It's not what happens to us. It's what we tell ourselves about what happens to us that makes the difference.

When we experience the loss of someone we love, we are left with a deep pain. We are also left with a story that we tell ourselves and others about our loss. That story will change as we work through our grief. Eventually our story will either keep us paralyzed and stuck in grief, or will empower us to move on with our lives.

Initially, it is natural that our story of loss be filled with negative emotions and the drama that often surrounds those emotions:

Anger: "This shouldn't be happening to me! This is not fair!"

Guilt: "I should have spent more time with him. I should have been there for her."

Fear: "How will I survive now that he's gone? How can I stand the loneliness?"

The more drama and negative emotion we have within our story of loss, the more difficult it is to move beyond our grief. We need to work through each negative emotion, but then, as soon as possible, we need to reframe our story so that it empowers us and assists us in moving on with our lives.

The steps in reframing our story are these:

1. Remove the drama and admit the emotion. It is better to say "I am angry!" than to say "This isn't fair!" or "This should not be happening!" When we admit anger or

➤

guilt or fear, without the dramatic embellishments, it is easier to work through these emotions.

2. Remove the drama and emotion, and admit the pain. Moving beyond the negative emotions and admitting the deep pain of our loss is healthy and healing—to expose and express and truly be with the experience of the pure pain of our loss. We can now say: "I feel pain!"

3. Celebrate the person, the gift, and the opportunity within our situation. We can reframe the story to say "I'm grateful that this wonderful person was in my life for as long as he/she was," or "Now that my life has changed, I welcome opportunities to learn and grow and be of service to others in many new and positive ways. I am grateful for the opportunities that reveal themselves now and in the future."

We usually need to take these steps one at a time, over time. Reframing our story step by step is a wonderful tool for moving beyond the paralysis of our grief and moving on with our lives.

New Blossoms

"When spring comes, the grass grows by itself."
FROM THE TAO TE CHING

At the first dance class I taught after Robert's death, Juanita—a feisty eighty-year-old woman, herself a widow—watched me across the room and said matter-of-factly, "Joan, you look terrible!"

The class gasped, but I smiled at the comic relief of her honesty. I'm sure I did look terrible—eyes red and glassy, face swollen from crying, body slumped from the weight of losing my dearest love. "But you'll look good again," she assured me. This time the class joined me in laughter.

I thought I could get through my grief as long as I could keep teaching my line-dance classes. That's where Robert and I met and danced our whole seven years together. It was a place of joy for us, and it remained a refuge and a bit of relief from the grief after he died. I would cry all day, then pull myself together an hour before class, and focus mind and body on teaching my dance class.

Then one day, two and a half months after Robert died, I realized I could not stop crying in time to teach my class that evening. I phoned my doctor's office, sobbing, asking for help. My doctor started me on an antidepressant for "situational depression" (a term I hadn't known, but it fit) and set me up to see a therapist. I also wrote in my journal, talked to hospice counselors, participated in support groups, read books about grief—I did it all. The grief journey became my day job. I gave myself the gift of a year to experience my grief fully, without any responsibilities except keeping myself as healthy as I could manage, teaching my dance classes, and feeding my cat. I put the book I had started—this one—on hold.

During the most extreme grief, the antidepressant didn't kill the pain or lift the fog, but it dulled the knife's sharpness and lightened the darkness enough that I could function a little—not enough to write this book, but I was able to teach my classes and keep up with my blog to stay in touch with my readers. I still felt like I was bicycling through peanut butter, but at least the elephant had stopped kicking me in the chest.

For the first few months, the combination of grief and antidepressant buried my sex drive. I didn't even have sex with myself. I told my therapist, "I know I should keep my sexual self alive through self-pleasuring, but it just seems like too much trouble. I wonder if it will even still work."

"If you have a vibrator," she said, "it will still work."

She was right.

But sex beyond self-pleasure was another issue entirely. Friends and even curious readers would ask, "Can you see yourself dating again, getting in a relationship again, having sex again?"

At first, I said no. I had found and lost my great love—no one could follow that. I had a social life: teaching dance, making walking and dinner dates with friends, both male and female. I was still interested in sex, but more as a writer and sex educator than in my personal life.

Then, amazingly, about six months into my grieving, I started to feel stirrings. I found myself feeling turned on by men who radiated that enticing combination of sexuality and gentleness. I marveled at feeling the urge again. We human beings are amazingly resilient.

I had a dream at that time that I was responding sexually to a fully dressed, sexy man who was pressing his aroused self against me. I awoke, excited and filled with wonder. "I'm still alive!" I said aloud.

Sure enough, many months later, Juanita said to me, "You look really good. You're feeling better. I told you!" We don't get over grief, we get through it. I don't miss Robert less, but somehow life is manageable again, and I'm capable of joy and laughter.

Although I couldn't imagine this at first, I'll have a lover again, and it will be good. I won't try to replace the love I shared with Robert—impossible—but there's a resiliency, a joy bubbling up that makes me feel vibrant and alive. Nurturing my sexual and loving self is a part of being fully alive that I will embrace, when it's time.

But everyone grieves and heals differently. Some jump quickly into a new relationship; others never do. Most date again, and many find new loves. Some never feel they're ready. As grief counselors assured me, whatever you're feeling is normal. Whatever you're doing about it—or not doing about it—is normal. Feeling sexy is normal. Not feeling sexy is normal. Not knowing what you feel is normal.

How did others reclaim their sexuality after losing their beloved partners? Their stories offer hope and proof of our amazing resilience. As raw as our grief is, and as isolated and stricken as we may feel, we can find solace in learning how others coped and found joy again.

Grief and Healing

Not all the people in this chapter wanted another sexual relationship, even years later. There is no right or wrong way, and no official time period that marks the end of grief or the beginning of a time for new relationships. Each person's experience is unique, as you'll see in these stories.

CHLOE, AGE 70

My husband died of a brain tumor after forty years together. After he died, I felt like a zombie. I did what I had to do without much feeling. I never broke down or grieved until a week or two after the funeral. Yet I felt sexual almost immediately. I sort of panicked and masturbated frequently, three times a week. I did not want to lose that part of my life too. I watched videos and used my vibrator.

Three months after my husband died, I took my rings off. That very day, an old friend I had feelings for a long time ago came over, and we had sex. It felt so good. We both desired each other, and it has not stopped since. We are not married but have lived together for eight years, and we are very happy with this type of relationship. Funny, when we first got together, I said, "This will not last three weeks," and look at us now. We make love two to three times a week.

What is normal for one couple is not necessary normal for another. Our age group still tends to live by certain guidelines, which are absolute poppycock. I'm all for living my life fully. That includes a healthy sex life.

PETER, AGE 63

Diane and I moved in together a few months after our first date. We were together for thirty-three years. We were always cuddling and kissing, and I rarely passed behind her without kissing the back of her neck.

Sex was frequent and hot at first. Diane took to oral sex enthusiastically, and we did a little Polaroid play. Taking photographs was an enormous source of stimulation for me. It helped both of us shed our inhibitions. I still have the photographs, and they are a source of great joy and nostalgia. Three children and one vasectomy later, sex became less central to our lives, although it was still satisfying and varied.

I had my first bout with prostate cancer in 2001, with radiation following. I gradually became able to have an erection again, but I remember masturbating alone a couple of times, and I ejaculated a lot of blood. From then on, my sperm became clear and sticky, and this inhibited me from orgasm with Diane, as it seemed most unpleasant to me.

We still engaged in sexual activity. We began with a nice long shower, with genital and general body caressing, and sometimes penetration without an orgasm on my part. Diane would often come this way, followed by oral sex and then intercourse in the bedroom.

The last time we had intercourse was October 2004. After that, she said, "I'm just not interested anymore." We were still affectionate and loving, but I accepted that physical sex would never happen again.

Diane was diagnosed with cancer of the pancreas in 2006. Unfortunately, the cancer had spread too far to be treatable. I resigned from my job, and Diane and I spent all our time together for the last year of her life. Diane and I grieved together for a year before she died, a privilege that very few people are blessed with. I was prepared for her death and knew that there would be a life ahead. If her death had been sudden, I think I would have fallen to pieces.

I haven't been in a sexual relationship since Diane died. I have done some Internet dating, and one relationship led to an evening of heavy petting, but otherwise, they've all been sexless. Despite a loss of libido from my prostate-cancer treatment, I am still interested in developing a sensual relationship with a partner. I'm reasonably confident that time, patience, and care will help me to become erect, and now that I've read *Better Than I Ever Expected*, I understand that an erection is not the sine qua non of good sex over sixty. This was a real eye-opener for me. I do look forward to making new friends, and I dearly hope that one of them will blossom into a sexual relationship.

SHMILY, AGE 69

I was married at twenty-one and was a virgin on my wedding night. I changed into my peignoir set in the bathroom and slipped into bed. My new husband, naked, quickly joined me—and quickly finished. Afterward, my thought was, "Is that all there is?" I did not want to make him feel inadequate, so I did not let him know how disappointed I was.

With more experience, things began to work like they should, and the years began to roll. We had a child, we worked, we played, we loved, we grew. As he aged, he became a considerate lover, and our sex was ever so much better. He made sure that I was receiving what I wanted.

We had fourteen wonderful years of retirement together. As physical ailments came along, we never had a problem in finding "a way." He would tease me, "Ma, some day you will miss me and realize how good a hard man is to find!" Oh, how right he was! That day is here. He passed away almost three years ago.

On the night that he passed, we went to bed together and cuddled. He got up saying he did not feel good. Then he said, "I'm having trouble breathing." I had been on oxygen for six years, so I got my portable oxygen and put it on him. He had to go to the bathroom and carried the oxygen in with him. He wasn't in there a minute when I heard a crash. I dialed 911, and the EMTs worked a long time on him, but it was useless. He was gone.

After such a strong bond and wonderful marriage, I still to this day cannot imagine I would be able to have a male lover, as much as I miss the sex. I guess I truly am a one-man woman. I have experimented with sex toys. It sure is hard work alone. I am capable of satisfying my physical needs, but it feels so lacking in the emotional and sharing aspects of lovemaking.

I have been considering having a female lover. It strikes me as a better possibility. While married, I never had any thoughts along these lines. Now I wonder if the thought of replacing him with another man is so abhorrent to me that I would welcome a female lover instead.

CHERYL, AGE 78

My husband and I were together forty-six years. Our sex life blossomed after the kids were grown. We could fool around on the living-room couch, not just in the bedroom. Once in a while we would rent a soft-core film and have our own private orgy—sex more than once in the course of an evening, then again in the early morning.

However, my husband was a drinker, and eventually his use of alcohol affected his ability to have intercourse. He tried Viagra, but it didn't help. His doctor ordered a pump-type device, which worked for a while. Later, his alcohol use and age were too much for the device to handle, but we didn't give up on our sex life. We enjoyed foreplay and manual stimulation. We were still enjoying sex in the best ways we could when he passed away of a heart attack at age seventy-four.

I held nightly conversations with him after he died. I slept on his side of the bed, on his pillow, and wore one of his T-shirts. I had a bench erected for him; it overlooks the ocean, and I go there to talk to him often.

I met a gentleman I was interested in spending time with, but I worried about what would happen if he wanted a sexual relationship. I didn't want to become sexually involved, both because of my strong faith—which does not condone sex without marriage—and because it was too soon. As it turned out, he had lost his ability to perform and was grateful that I didn't expect sex from him.

I do engage in solo sex, occasionally. I decided that as long as I consider it to be a visit with my husband and visualize him with me, it is a good thing.

I find sensuality in other things: dancing to salsa music, swimming, soaking in the sun, savoring a sinful dessert. My Zumba dance classes, which involve sensual hip movements, help me to express and release my sensuality. When my eight-year-old grandson stays overnight, he hugs and kisses me and strokes my face while I'm reading a bedtime story. If I close my eyes, I can almost feel the touch of my late husband. I wake up feeling grateful every day for all that I have.

ESTHER, AGE 63

Sex with my husband was twenty minutes of foreplay and shoot for the finish. Intimacy was long gone before he died. I was busy raising two boys, so I put it out of my mind. Now, fifteen years later, I'm dealing with diminished vaginal-tissue elasticity, and this presents a real challenge.

My husband died a year and a half ago. I wasn't looking for love, but in reaching out to a friend after the loss of his wife, a close friendship developed.

Getting sexual again has been a real trip. But I've done it, largely with the help from *Better Than I Ever Expected* and Joan's blog, with its wonderful information and links. These opened the doors to a new world of pleasure, confidence, and courage. Judith Sills's book, *Getting Naked Again*, gave me the final push. She suggested having a friend "mentor" your reentry into getting naked again.

So that's what I did. I asked this dear friend to help me in this tremendous step. We had been dating for a few months, very cautiously, as he is a more recent widower and not ready for any new relationship. This mentoring idea appealed to him.

We clarified just what we were doing and why. We shared our feelings, our limitations, and our fears. I asked that we use condoms or get tested for STDs. It was an amazingly honest and open sharing.

Once we knew these intimate details about each other, the whole experience was positive—a wonderful three hours. We both enjoyed it so much that we have continued the relationship.

We focus on total-body sex, delighting in caressing, massaging, kissing, licking. We bring each other to climax with our hands and mouths after hours of pleasuring. After a month of wonderful sexual sharing, he suddenly said he was having trouble dealing with the new feelings and relationship while remembering the lost one. We backed off the sex, and continued a close and loving friendship, to allow him to work on his grief. Six weeks later, we slowly added touching back to our relationship. Now we are again comfortable sharing intimacy.

We communicate openly and comfortably about everything. I had never experienced oral sex before. Fortunately, my partner delights in pleasuring me this way. I also bought a vibrator and some black lingerie for the first time in my life. We hope that vaginal penetration is in our future.

MIRIAM, AGE 57

After my husband died, I spent a full year doing very little of life's demands—work, household chores—and instead gave my full attention to grieving the death of my husband. I'd been with him for twenty-eight years. I couldn't imagine being with anyone else.

When my interest did start to warm to the idea of being in love again, honest to God, I truly wondered if sex was a transferable skill! I'd only had one sex partner for twenty-eight years, and I thought, *Does this stuff work with anyone else?* Intellectually, I knew it was a ridiculous question. But on a gut and heart level, I couldn't imagine being comfortable sexually with someone else. What if the next guy doesn't have such deep brown eyes to gaze into? What if his lips don't fit with mine like my husband's did?

Then it happened, more than a year after my husband's death. What a surprise—sex *is* a transferable skill! There was this incredibly poignant moment when I first made love with a new man. While we kissed, I felt his collar bones in the palms of my hands. I was lying rib-to-rib with him. The full contact of our skin felt glorious. I started to cry.

I love the visceral, I'm-loving-you-through-my-five-senses bonding that happens between lovers. That kind of connection with my husband was lost forever when he died. Even though I still remembered him, told stories about him, and felt his presence in my life, that raw, lovely, passionate touch-feast was *gone*.

Now I was with a new man I loved, and I had that visceral connection again. It was fantastic. Those first few times with him, I cried tears of loss and tears of joy. It was a spiritual experience—a hyperawareness and reminder to savor the touch of my lover because of the knowledge of our mortality.

He helped me "metabolize" some remaining grief through my transition to a new life. After two years together, we are no longer lovers. But I'm thankful for our sweet sharing during such an important time.

MIKE, AGE 52

I was forty-seven when I lost my soul mate, Larry, age seventy. We had been together twenty-four years and had already together survived his heart bypass surgery and recovery. One St. Patrick's Day, we attended a party and danced wildly. The next day, Larry was vomiting and twisting in pain. His bladder-cancer diagnosis was a huge blow to both of us.

As Larry's illness and suffering worsened, I had ambivalent feelings. As much as I adored Larry, part of me was seeing my worst nightmare becoming reality—being a caregiver to a slowly dying person, and depleting all my emotional, physical, and financial resources along the way.

I was meditating when I heard a voice telling me Larry was going to die within a year, although the doctors had predicted five to ten years. What would I do if I knew that Larry had less than a year to live? I would be more loving, spend more time with him, spend more money having fun together.

This was a very important decision, because the voice was right. We went on weekend trips, we meditated and prayed together, we talked. We continued to have a good sex life, despite the fact that Larry no longer had his prostate.

On our twenty-fourth anniversary, Larry wrote me a beautiful letter celebrating our love and leaving me with wonderful blessings for the rest of my life. He died a few weeks later. I was numb with grief, unable to sleep or cry. My sexual part, though, was excited, and my fantasy life went into overdrive. I craved someone to sleep with. I propositioned a friend, who turned me down. My sleeplessness and depression worsened. I was constantly sick. I saw a therapist and started taking Prozac, which did its magic. I was able to sleep and eat and was less sickly.

Three months after losing Larry, I started dating again. I had sex with a number of men—friends, new acquaintances, Internet dates. Each relationship started out sexy and comforting but never stayed that way.

After the one-year anniversary, I stopped taking Prozac and was doing fine. I enjoyed the freedom of single life. But what was I really looking for? I spent twenty-four years with a soul mate. Now I wanted a sexual fantasy.

I met Clive at a gay dance club. He was tall, radiant, with beautiful blue eyes—a dream come true. I just wanted to dance with him, afraid that such a hot man would not be interested in me. He was interested, and we began a three-year relationship that recently ended.

Five years after Larry died, I am happy again. I am dating, though I am not sure whether the ongoing presence of Larry in my life and the presence of my godchildren will leave me open for a full-fledged new relationship. I know that twenty-four years of a deep love is more than most people get during a lifetime.

BELINDA, AGE 78

My husband and I had been together for forty-six years when he died. Ours was a lusty, robust bonding of body and soul. He was a strong, passionate, street-smart guy. We worked together in a family business that became quite successful, and then we lost everything—three times. Our deep and abiding love grew stronger with every test.

Our sex life was sensual, tender, exciting, and frequent. But the last fourteen years of his life were a gradual decline due to health problems. Our affection only deepened.

He died after running out of oxygen one day when no one was home. I was so turned off from all the turmoil of his illness and death that I cannot remember any sexual stirrings until after a year and a half. I went dancing and met a man who fell for me—and I was attracted to him. I thought those feelings were permanently dead. But I was wrong, and I welcomed and explored them.

About twenty months after my husband died, I became sexual with this new man. There was real chemistry, for the first time in a very long time. He opened me up. He still does. We are not life partners. We are dancing partners and lovers. I have my life, he has his life, and we have our life together. We spend three nights a week together. It is a delightful arrangement.

17

Sensuality for Hire

Our Sacred Session may involve sensual, intimate, touch—unconditionally loving your body with sacred, sensual and erotic touch. . . . This touch may stimulate you and result in a climax of pleasure—however, the goal of orgasm is not the focus of the Sacred Session.

—SUNYATA, WWW.SUNYATASATCHITANANDA.COM

I READ SUNYATA'S WEBSITE over and over, pausing over these words. Then, on November 1, 2009, I wrote him this email.

Sunyata, I lost my beloved husband to cancer. I have been celibate for a year and a half, despite being a writer about sexuality. Although my toys enable me to keep my sexuality strong, I have been longing to be the recipient of a respectful, gentle, erotic massage with no body parts off-limits. Your Erotic Enrichment, as described on your website, seems to fit what I am seeking.

He emailed back, and then we had a phone conversation. We made an appointment for my sixty-sixth birthday.

Me? Hire someone I've never met to give me an "erotic massage," with every intention that it will lead to orgasm? Yes. I did it, I loved it, and it still brings a smile to my face and a tingle to my nether parts remembering it. (Now I'm really shocking my family.)

Brave? Maybe. Typical of me? Absolutely not—I had never done anything like this before. Foolhardy? It didn't seem so. He was recommended by someone I knew, and his website and client references seemed professional and impressive. Sure, a bad guy could construct an appealing website with convincing testimonials, but would a bad guy go to the trouble of claiming to be a Certified Tantric Healer, Reiki Master, and Universal Life Church Minister? Would a bad guy even know what these terms meant?

Isn't it a fantasy of ours—a pair of skilled hands focused on giving erotic pleasure, no reciprocation expected (or allowed), nonsleazy, all pleasure, orgasms included? I wasn't buying sex, Sunyata assured me. I wasn't buying any *outcome*. I was simply hiring his services. And if I happened to get carried away experiencing his services—these are my words, not his—every response would be accepted and celebrated.

I still missed Robert like crazy. I had been with Robert exclusively for our seven years together, and his face, hands, and body were the images that stirred my fantasy life when I aroused myself. I pictured Robert as he was through all but the last months of our relationship, vital and strong: a dancer's body, an artist's hands, a lover's smile. I imagined that he was the one touching me when I touched myself. I heard his murmurs of love. I saw his body responding to my touch. I felt his kiss.

And now I wondered: If another man were to touch me intimately, would I even be able to respond? Sunyata seemed a safe way to find out. I would pay his fee, lie on his massage table, and receive his full attention for two hours.

Sunyata started our session with a discussion, both of us fully clothed. (He would remain so—I would not.) He asked me questions and listened compassionately. He explained that he was offering his service to honor me, and it would not be reciprocal—it was not for his sexual pleasure, and his boundaries included not touching his genitals.

In other words, I was to get naked, climb on the table, relax, and receive.

It was bliss. I gave myself up to Sunyata's expert hands and floated on an ocean of gentle massage, culminating in crashing waves of pleasure. I laughed, I cried, I laughed again.

"You must love your job," I mumbled to Sunyata.

"I love my job," he said. I pictured him smiling, but I didn't manage to open my eyes to find out.

My birthday erotic massage from a gentle stranger changed something in me. It showed me that I was still a responsive, fully sexual woman, getting ready to emerge from the cocoon of mourning into reexperiencing life. I realized that one big reason I ended up on Sunyata's massage table was so that I could get ready to reenter the world.

Just the Sex, Please

Suppose you're not looking for an erotic massage with a spiritual bent, but full-on sex. If your fantasy runs to a handsome, debonair escort who will wine and dine you before helping you slip out of your dress, there are professional escort agencies. You pay your money, and a well-dressed hunk of man opens doors for you, laughs at your jokes, and shares fine dining (on your tab), with a separately negotiated fee if you and he agreed that a romp in your bed would be a nice finale to the evening.

But maybe you want to skip the evening on the town and go straight to wild sex that leaves you gasping?

When I read a few years ago that Heidi Fleiss was trying to open a brothel where women could come (so to speak) and be sexually serviced by alluring men, I thought that sounded like a great idea. Why not? I thought especially of women of my age and older who were not in relationships, didn't have buddies with benefits, and were not likely to pick up men for a casual encounter—but who would willingly pay for an hour or three of sexual pleasure, focused entirely on stimulating and satisfying *them*.

Although Fleiss encountered too many legal problems to open her Stud Farm, sexy men for hire are indeed available to women. And some of my female readers who were single or in dissatisfying marriages wrote me and described their experiences hiring pleasure providers. But would I advise women to do this, if they were so inclined? I didn't know, so I consulted Carol Queen, who—besides having a PhD in sexology and knowing everything about sex (both academic and nitty-gritty)—was once a sex worker and is the most sex-positive and nonjudgmental person I know. I emailed Carol the following.

> *Suppose a senior woman wants to hire a man for sex. Never mind erotic massage or Tantra—just excite her and give her body every pleasure she wants to experience. How does she find someone who will respect her and whatever agreement they make; do what she wants and no more; not scare her (unless she wants someone to scare her); and respect his own and her health enough to use barrier protection always? Craigslist? I'm sure the good ones are buried somewhere in there, but so are the men who rob or murder their clients. Male-escort agencies might seem a good way to go, but they're very expensive, and she might not have any interest in wining and dining. Any advice?*

Carol never backs away from a challenge. After reminding me that "paying for erotic services is illegal almost everywhere," she offered these suggestions.

ADVICE FROM AN EXPERT

For Women: Hiring Erotic Services

BY CAROL QUEEN, PHD

The real challenge here is that in most places—in the United States at least—there's no easy-to-find world of male providers for female clients. In some locales, you may need to call escort agencies that advertise women for male clients and find out whether they have guys on staff. In some places, males-for-men agencies or classified ads in the gay newspaper will yield bisexual men.

How to negotiate: If the woman has ever had the opportunity to say exactly what she wants, it's now. She's paying for a service! She should put it all out there, including safer-sex expectations—and she should always insist on safer sex. On the other hand, many pros and agencies will not allow explicit discussion on the phone. It's how they prevent themselves from getting set up.

Yes, there is some danger, but probably not more than you'd face when simply cruising Craigslist for action. Always tell a trusted friend that you are going off on an adventure and that you will call at an appointed time—then make that call. Instruct your friend to get help if you don't call. This is called a "silent alarm." It works best when you tell your date right up front that someone is expecting a call from you and knows

➤

where you are. If you set this up, you *must* make the call, even if you are in a postcoital haze.

Don't drink or otherwise indulge too much with an unknown partner—keep your wits and intuition sharp enough to know when you do and don't feel safe. And don't engage in bondage in this situation. If you want to explore bondage, there are parties you can attend that are set up for this purpose, and where you'll be safe.

CLAIRE, AGE 56

I was married, but our marriage had become celibate. I masturbated but felt unsatisfied. I didn't want an affair, because I loved my husband and family, but I needed more. I turned to the Internet, Googled "SF Bay Area male escort," and browsed the ads. One of the escorts was a very handsome man named Bernardo. Our meeting was a turning point in my life.

Bernardo was even more attractive than in his photos. He closed the room shades, lit candles, set up his massage table, and had me lie down. He began with a wonderful massage, then began to caress my breasts, moving his hands down my body. He made love to me with his fingers and lips until I climaxed over and over. At age forty-nine, I had never been attended to in such a way by a lover.

As he was ministering to me, I could see his erection pressing against his sexy satin shorts. "It's okay to touch," he said. Quickly we moved to the bed, and I experienced the best sex I ever had.

We began meeting at least once a month, and this went on for years. The $100 fee, plus the cost of a hotel room, was a stretch financially, but I sacrificed in other areas to budget these encounters—they were that important to me. After about six months, he asked that I no longer pay him, telling me that he received as much joy and comfort from the relationship as I did. He allowed me to be comfortable with any form of sexual pleasure I desired: toys, fantastic anal sex, and orgasm after orgasm for both of us.

Before Bernardo, I used sex for control, to exchange for something. In college—though I could have earned top grades with my intellect—I exchanged blow jobs with my professors for A's. Sex was a commodity.

In my marriage, I had sex primarily to please my husband. It was hardly ever enjoyable or intimate—just a quick release for him only. He was a selfish lover, never using his fingers or engaging in oral sex unless it was me going down on him. I asked him to kiss me, and his reply was "Men don't kiss their wives like that."

With Bernardo, I learned to experience sex for pure pleasure. It's been life-changing.

Bernardo and I continue to see each other today—sometimes just for dinner, most times for passionate, hot sex as lovers, but not as a prostitute and his "jane." Sometimes we just sleep in each other's arms. Other times, we are like two animals devouring each other.

As I write this, I am also text messaging Bernardo to see if he wants to spend time together tonight.

MARK, AGE 54

I turned to sex-for-hire after my wife made it clear that she did not enjoy sex anymore. Our marriage became celibate. I was faced with stark choices:

1. remain celibate (too difficult, and, frankly, I didn't see why I should)

2. leave my wife and find someone else (not an option; I love my wife and adore our children)

3. have an affair

4. pay for sex

This last one seemed the "least bad" option. I reasoned with myself that as it was just sex, an animal act, I was not being emotionally unfaithful.

Certainly my ego would be stroked more by having an affair. I would know that the person is doing it because she finds me attractive, rather than just being paid. However, the risk of emotional attachment by one or both of us is great. I had one real affair. It was disastrous emotionally. She became attached, and I ran away. I honestly believe that hiring sex is not threatening to my marriage. Having an affair is.

Hiring sex is a surprisingly honest transaction. The provider and I both know why we are together. To find sexual providers, I tried researching various review sites, like The Erotic Review (www.theeroticreview.com), but these sites are of limited use. I want to ask the reviewer, "Yes, but are you like me? Are you looking for the same things I am?" A thirty-year-old wants something very different from a fifty-year-old, so reading that a particular provider is good at x, y, or z does not paint the picture that I want. I find word-of-mouth recommendation to be more reliable.

When I started hiring escorts, I was drawn to sexual beauty and youth. I soon found that sex with these women was not particularly sexually fulfilling—rather like having a McDonald's when you're hungry. I am attracted to intelligent, witty women, often demonstrated in their online blogs. Once I have found one, I look to see who else is on her blogroll. I have never had a bad experience following this path.

If you, like me, are seeking to fill in the bits that are missing from your marriage and not to end your marriage, you need to be discrete. Do not take stupid risks. Be honest with yourself. What are you looking to find in a commercial sexual relationship? Is it just sexual release? Someone who will listen to you without criticism? Emotional fulfilment? A confidante? One escort described her job to me as being more "emotion worker" than "sex worker."

There is absolutely no point in lying to a sex worker about what you want from the engagement. They do not sell their bodies, they sell a service. Make sure you find someone who will provide the service you are looking for.

From the Providers

I wondered what motivates practitioners, especially those over fifty. Are they just performing a service, doing their job? Is this a mission to give everyone the sensual experiences they desire, regardless of age, appearance, relationship status? Do they feel a spiritual calling? Are they turned on? Would they talk to me candidly?

Although I got different answers to the first questions, the last one received a resounding "Yes!" Some of the practitioners were skittish about revealing their identity; others had websites with contact information and testimonials. I didn't choose to interview any providers that struck me personally as sleazy—the ones pushing their breasts, tongues, or erections into the camera, or bragging about cup-size or penis length. If that's your cup of cocoa, you can find those on your own.

Instead, I chose a few practitioners who had reasons for providing their services besides earning a good hourly rate; who respected their clients and were proud of how happy these clients were after a session. Here are a few of their stories.

EVELYNN, SEXUAL ENERGY PROFESSIONAL, AGE 65

I consider my sexual energy to be my life. I have come to love my body, and I have embraced my "wild older woman," as well as my "wise older woman."

In my late forties I noticed that my desire was getting more intense and more focused on quality versus quantity. I began practicing Tantra and discovered a whole new awareness of orgasmic energy as my life force. It continues to become more intense the older I get. It's my fountain of youth.

Twelve years ago, I stepped into my role as a sexual energy professional. Accepting that first client who walked through my door was exhilarating and scary all at once. I have never regretted my decision.

I often work in the nude, and I touch genitals. My focus is on helping my client integrate his/her genitals back into the good graces of his/her body and soul. I am trained as a sexological bodyworker, as well as other somatic modalities that incorporate touch of the entire body. What I do is often considered against the law. However, I never charge a fee—those who visit me donate to my sanctuary, my temple. What I do is not against my laws.

Many who seek my counsel are over fifty and over sixty. I work with Parkinson's patients, abuse survivors, prostate-cancer survivors, and those who suffer from perceived erectile dysfunction. My teachings get down to the nitty-gritty of showing my students how to get back into understanding how their bodies work with their energies.

I have been coloring outside the lines for many years. The rewards to those I see are far more real to me than the risk of crossing over sexually repressive boundaries. A large underground of somatic healers continues to be amazed at the power of sexual energy to heal. We consider ourselves "powerful outlaws."

—*Visit EveLynn's website at www.awakeningbody.com.*

SUNYATA SATCHITANANDA, DAKA, TANTRIC HEALER, REIKI MASTER, AGE 50

My private sessions create a safe opportunity for men and women of all adult ages to enhance, explore, and expand an underserved aspect of life: sensual touch needs. Often my clients are women who are celibate—out of circumstance or conscience—yet recognize their need for sensual touch. A sexual healer (Daka) skillfully nurtures the human need of intimate, sensual touch.

Regardless of being touched sensually by a "stranger," there is no intention for a personal, romantic relationship, and no reciprocal touch. My sexual desire or gratification does not enter the space of our sacred session. I focus on being present with your desire and what wants to release or be revealed. Your sexual body receives attention and is given nurturing and healing engagement that sponsors well-being and fulfillment.

It can be difficult to find a Daka locally; normally they don't openly advertise their services due to cultural and legal hassles. The Internet provides some assistance. Some local Tantra educators are also skilled Dakas. I recommend interviewing the prospective practitioner, asking about experience and training, and trusting your intuition about suitability and compatibility. Get testimonials and references if possible.

—*Visit Sunyata's website at www.sunyatasatchitananda.com*

HERCULES, THERAPEUTIC SENSUAL MASSAGE THERAPIST, AGE 40

I have worked as a massage therapist for over twenty years. I never crossed the line between traditional massage and sensual massage until six years ago. I was approached by a regular client, who asked if I would give her a more sensual massage, including massaging her vulva to orgasm. She found massage to be very sensual, intimate, and arousing. She was disgruntled that there were places for men to get massage with orgasmic release but not a safe and trustworthy place for women.

Her request seemed reasonable. Personally, I had experienced massages with release, and I could see the therapeutic value. So I did a session for her, and she loved it. She told her best friend, and this is how I began to develop my Therapeutic Sensual Massage, a practice that is professional but not clinical, sensual but not sleazy.

Therapeutic Sensual Massage focuses on the whole body, from scalp to toes and everything in between, including genitals. I combine the healing aspect of massage with the sensuality aspect. I am working to release the body from tension, pain, and stress. Eventually we work toward the ultimate release of orgasm. When you get a wonderful massage, you feel as if energy is just flowing off of you, but when it includes the release of an orgasm, you feel as if the energy is flowing from the inner core of you as well.

—*Learn more about Hercules at www.thepleasurecoach.org.*

LILY, EROTIC MASSEUSE, AGE 58

I have been doing sensual massage for seven years, after burning out on a long career in advertising. My work keeps me feeling sexy, juicy, and desirable. By learning how to provide a better service for my clients, I have expanded the boundaries of my own sexuality.

The prevailing theme of my sessions is that the client's cock is the guest of honor. I like to intermix a relaxing massage with abundant teasing. I start with a slow sensuous back massage with some teasing, tickling of the balls, draping my body across his back, running my fingers across his butt, caressing his inner thighs.

Eventually I focus my attention exclusively on his genital area. I have learned from this work that a man's first relationship is with his penis, his best friend who is always with him and always demanding. As a woman who pampers and cherishes his friend, I am much appreciated.

I've been told I have great hands: sensuous, curious, gentle, yet purposeful. They caress, stroke, tickle, and titillate. They are hands on a mission to pamper and bring that cock to its ultimate bliss. All my clients leave happy, and over the years, I've built up a healthy repeat business.

The downside is that the nature of my work makes it impossible for me to be in an intimate relationship myself. Most men don't have a strong enough ego for it. So I am on the alert for an exit strategy. When I do leave this work and start a new life with a relationship, I will do it with full knowledge that honoring and doting over a man's best friend is an important way to keep him happy and to keep me beautiful and sexy, in his eyes, forever.

18

DWO: Dating While Old(er)

S O HOW DO you meet someone, at our age? Many find their matches on online dating sites. Personally, I advocate doing the social and educational activities that you really enjoy, and you'll meet people who enjoy what you do. I wanted a man who enjoyed dancing as much as I do, so I spent my free time social dancing. I figured that the man of my dreams wouldn't be sitting home reading the personals ads or going online, but would be out (duh!) dancing.

I was right. I met the love of my life when he wandered into my very own line dancing class. He had recently moved to the area and was looking for a place to dance. He found more than he expected.

I recount our love story in *Better Than I Ever Expected*—it was the reason I wrote that book. Our meeting illustrates why I recommend doing what you love, and how you'll meet other people who match your interest. That's no guarantee of true love, but if you're excited about an activity and wish you could share it with someone, try the direct route. Also, if you're doing what you enjoy, you project a different kind of joy, energy, and attractiveness compared to going somewhere with the sole purpose of "meeting someone."

Desperation is easy to spot and a major turn-off. The more self-sufficient we are, the more we enjoy our own company, the more we know what we have to give, the better we can share our love with another person. Potential mates sense that kind of self-assurance and are drawn to someone whose life is already full and rewarding. Whether your mate comes along quickly or takes the long path getting to you, you'll enjoy yourself along the way. I think if you're open and happy with yourself, you may meet your mate anywhere.

But it's true: If you're reentering the dating world after decades, you may feel like there's some catching up to do. This chapter will help you navigate those changes. And if you want more, check out my blog, www.NakedAtOurAge.com, where I review many books about dating after age fifty.

KELLY, AGE 70

How do I know if I'm being too aggressive? Am I supposed to let the man set the pace and just hope for the best? The last thing in the world I want to do is to embarrass or humiliate or make him uncomfortable in any way, but how do I know the boundaries?

I would happily make love every night and probably every morning, too. I have such passionate responses that I feel vulnerable with someone I don't know very well, who might take advantage of the situation.

One guy would not rest until he got me into bed. Then—after *he* came—he had the nerve to say, "Gee, honey, you're still all tense and I don't quite know what to do about it." I looked at him and said, "Go home!" I made up my mind in 1987 that I'd do without rather than put up with the selfish men I kept finding. They wanted everything, but gave nothing.

Joan Responds

Kelly, it seems to me that any decision we made in 1987 is worth revisiting now, especially when it makes us unhappy! Personally, I don't find older men selfish at all. I love that older men have learned how to please a woman, and because their own hormones aren't pushing quickly to the goal of sex, they are as happy taking their time as we are.

Your story, though, made me wonder: How do you know ahead of time whether a partner will be sexually giving, or concentrate on her or his own pleasure to the exclusion of yours? Are there code words in an online profile that translate to "Your pleasure guaranteed or I won't expect mine"? Guess not.

I always feel more at ease with men who get along with ex-wives and ex-lovers and have close women friends. This says to me that they like and value women and are unlikely to be users. Of course, the better we know the man before sharing intimacy, the more likely we are to choose well, but that's a personal choice. I'm all for doing whatever you want, whenever and with whomever you want, as long as everyone involved is willing (including any partner who isn't present).

Cyberdating, Cybermating

I hear from many seniors who found love—and others who found sexy romps—using online dating sites. I asked Yolanda Turner to comment on how you can make the experience better, whichever site you land on.

Online Dating Tips for Seniors

BY YOLANDA TURNER, EDD

Are you reentering the dating world and a bit nervous? Relax and enjoy it. If you've made it to this age, you can handle the online dating arena. You'll find you have more freedom in what you look for and how you present yourself than when you dated the first time around.

Think of yourself as the interviewer, not the interviewee. What type of person do you want to spend time with? Stop wondering if you are good enough for them. Ask yourself what *you* want to invite into *your* life.

What do you like about yourself? What do other people like about you? Put those qualities in your profile. Be honest, and stay positive in your description. Put up pictures that look like you—no photos from fifteen years or thirty pounds ago. Use a close up of your face, plus one or two in different environments. Use pictures to let people get to know you.

Do not look for your "soul mate" or say that in your profile. Online dating is a way to meet interesting, different people who can open up new areas of life to you. Look for a companion with whom to do fun things. Then see what happens.

If you describe the person you are looking for in your profile, only include the deal breakers—"must like dogs," "nonsmoker," whatever is essential to you. Describe the types of people you enjoy, not what you're "looking for in a mate." You'll be surprised at the multitude of experiences that will open up if you say "Why not?" to the idea of dating someone you might never have considered before.

➤

> Write a "first response" template letter that includes more specific information about you than is in your profile; you can send this as a "hello" to someone with an appealing profile. You can also copy and paste portions of this template when someone contacts you and you want to respond. Also create a polite "No, but thank you" template letter for people you are not interested in who contact you. Include a short, personal line specific to that person.

Always talk on the phone before you actually meet someone in person. Be cautious if someone can only talk at very specific times or can't talk in the evening. A married person hiding that fact will be confined to certain times to talk, and often won't want you to call. Single people will be much more available.

Ask open questions that will give you insight into who they are now, and who they were in the past. (The best question anyone ever asked me was "What was the biggest thing you learned from your divorce?")

Always date more than one person from the Internet at a time. You're not getting married—you're dating. If someone you are interested in turns out not to be the person you'd hoped, keep looking, and keep dating.

MIRIAM, AGE 57

I've been on four online dating sites since becoming single again. In the early months it was great to get in several repetitions of talking on the phone, meeting for coffee, and learning how to navigate this world of meeting strangers for potential relationships. I haven't met anyone I want to have a relationship with. But it has been a great way to tiptoe my way back to dating.

REDHAWK, AGE 62

I think fear of growing old without a lover inhibits gay men from embracing their aging. Online sites have been dissatisfying because I'm not just looking for sex—I'm looking for a relationship with similar men. I want a man my age who is grounded, emotionally literate and available, honest, able to communicate, self-aware, comfortable in his own sexuality, and willing and able to be vulnerable and adventuresome. Venues for finding this kind of relationship are almost nonexistent for gay men.

PETER, AGE 63

I'd like to know where all the sensual senior women are. I've joined several Internet dating sites and never encountered anyone who even remotely resembles any of the women in *Better Than I Ever Expected*. On one site, the profiles list so many "must-not's" that I sometimes wonder if there is anything they do want.

Joan Responds

Peter, the sensual senior women are all around you. They probably won't reveal that right away, though—they usually want to know that you value them as people and enjoy them as companions before they let their sensuality show. However, if someone lists more "must not's" than "want's," move on to another profile or another site. You might ask a close (and honest!) woman friend to read your profile and give you feedback about whether your most appealing qualities are showing.

The Scoop on Online Dating: A Woman's View

One of the most entertaining projects I started on my blog was a collaboration with Becka, who became my intrepid Internet dating reporter. This compilation of her experiences and tips will nudge you to share the adventure.

BECKA, AGE 70

Trying to decode the mystique of the Internet dating scene is like being lost in the middle of a Dan Brown book. "What does it all mean?" you ask yourself. These tips, which are based on my experience, should minimize the pain and maximize the delight.

Wading into the Senior Internet Dating Pool

There you are, filling out the questionnaire, and you lie. It can't be helped. Everybody lies. There are things that are just too personal and intimate to put out there on a website for the world to see. You are not providing a complete picture. Neither is anyone else.

Does he describe himself as "old-fashioned"? That's code for "I want a woman without any needs of her own, whose biggest joy is seeing to my every wish."

A woman who describes herself as having "a few extra pounds" can be trusted. She is probably ten pounds overweight or her perfect weight. A man, however, can be three hundred pounds overweight and use that phrase without blushing.

Too Many Men, Too Little Time, Not Enough Memory

The slew of responses I got was overwhelming. I winnowed and winnowed, trying to separate the wheat from the chaff. Here's why I rejected some of my "matches."

- Leo wrote that he was looking for a "soul mate to love forever" and then mentioned that his dog had passed away and "no one can replace that void."

- Alex, who's 5' 3" and makes less than $20,000 a year, thought I should know that he "reads women's magazines to study the opposition."

- Donald said, "I am a smoker, earn under $12,000, drink a little, am passive and submissive, and am looking for a woman who will finish the job my mother and sister started, when I was a kid, of turning me into a full female."

Becka Has Three Dates

You will learn a lot about yourself on this journey. I learned I liked a sense of humor, but sometimes lacked one myself. It took awhile for me to realize that Joe was joking when he wrote, "She must be breathing. If she's not breathing, the whole deal is off." Joe became Date No. 1. He makes me laugh.

I learned I am a risk taker. When Bill would not give additional information until I revealed something of myself, I complained. He wrote, "Aw, why wouldn't you want some mystery?" Bill became Date No. 2. We met at a local diner, and each of us wore something from Star Wars, so we'd recognize the other. (Now you know I'm a geek.)

My favorite is Steve, Date No. 3. He offered to cook for me, massage my feet, and "wander through the woods together, armed only with a camera." He suggested meeting at a hiking-club event. I felt safe and knew I'd have a good time, even if we didn't hit it off.

There are fabulous times to be had with wonderful people! You need two senses: "common sense" and "sense of adventure." "Sixth sense" doesn't hurt either. My three men are in a photo finish for my heart.

You are going to get a lot of inquiries. About 90 percent of them will not fit you, and you must reject them. But oh, those remaining 10 percent! Fabulous smiles, lots of charm, skills, personality plus, humble, sweet. Half of them will reject you. But that still leaves a dozen or two "possibles." And as my supportive friend Gloria said, "Becka, nobody's perfect, especially you."

—*In "real life," Becka is a Visionary artist in Maine and is still seeing Steve.*

Worst First Dates

Sometimes you just have to laugh at dating. Sherry Halperin filled a book with her dating disasters in her hilarious *Rescue Me, He's Wearing a Moose Hat: And 40 Other Dates after 50*. I asked my interviewees and blog readers about their worst first dates as seniors: What happened that let them know they'd rather sit alone with their cat than see this person again? (You never make any of these mistakes, right?)

- "He spent the entire dinner complaining about his ex. He went on and on about how women expected men to take charge of everything, pay for everything, yada, yada, yada."

- "I lived in the heart of the gay community in a very gay-friendly city. Mr. Bible Thumper declared, when he saw two men holding hands, 'Homosexuality is an abomination against God!' Being an agnostic and the sister of a late-in-life lesbian, I asked him what difference did it make to him? How is it any skin off his nose? 'I shouldn't have to be subjected to it,' he said. Oh brother."

- "I went to a paid dating service and had a date with a man who brought photos of his many possessions. It was pitiful."

- "This guy seemed literate and sane in our email conversations. He spent the first thirty minutes of our coffee date describing his medical problems in detail—his two heart bypasses and all his numbers: blood pressure, cholesterol, on and on. Finally, he took an interest in me by brightly asking, 'And what about you? What are *your* health problems?'"

- "He wore slippers. Enough said."

Michele Cauch, Executive Director of Sage*Health* Network, offers these simple guidelines for how to act on a first date: "Don't embarrass yourself, don't offend others, look nice, and smell good."

Women Seeking Women

Women seeking women are turning to Internet dating, and they too are quick to notice that online dating sites draw all kinds of hopefuls—from your perfect love match to predators and lost souls who would make your life a living hell if you got involved, as Irene discovered. Her story is followed by some great tips from psychologist Glenda Corwin for "weeding out the nuts" and recognizing the warning signs of troubled people with emotional problems. Although Dr. Corwin addresses her tips to women seeking women, they are tremendously useful to anyone in the world of online dating.

IRENE, AGE 50

I always knew I was attracted to women, but I married because of society's stigma. I was married for twenty years. It was hard to hide my feelings. We went out, and I looked at the girls like he did. I had dreams of having sex with women. At times I woke up having an orgasm, wondering if my husband knew what was going on. I never cheated on him, although I thought about it many times. Toward the end of our marriage, he said he always knew that I was, as he called it, "a fucking dyke."

I came out in 1993 and have been with seven girls, three long-term. My last girlfriend left me with only a two-day notice. I was devastated and thought I would never find someone again. My self-esteem was very low for a long time.

I started online dating to meet new people. I've had several dates, and I'm still out there looking. My problem is finding someone as sexual as I am. I think the older I get, the better sex gets. Just because we get older, we are not dead in the bed, and we still enjoy being stimulated. I love the touch and feel of a woman who is so soft she makes you melt. I've always been attracted to younger girls, thirty-five to fifty, and that's what I seem to attract.

Being intimate with someone new is scary. I try not to talk about my needs until I get to know someone. Once the jitters are gone and I feel comfortable, I will tell her what I want.

You have to search for the right girl and weed out the nuts. Weeding out the crazy ones who want to marry you after the first week can be frustrating. I recently went through this. She was a very nice lady who I thought could be the one. After one week she was questioning how much I drank, who I was having dinner with, and why wasn't I in love with her yet. She told me she was in love with me the day she met me.

Watching for Warning Signs

BY GLENDA CORWIN, PHD

I've talked with dozens of women who've met wonderful friends online, and a few who have met lovers and partners. It's a great avenue, but keep it realistic. You can't tell from words and photos if she's that warm woman you're looking for.

The best predictor of future behavior is past history. If she volunteers that she's been in a psychiatric hospital, or has been arrested for drunk driving, find out what happened next. Did she get better? Stop drinking? Go to therapy? Join a support network? Good people can recover from bad problems—if they are willing to do the work it takes. If not, be kind and compassionate, and be wise—stay away.

Most women don't volunteer such blatant information immediately, so listen for more subtle cues. If she says she goes to therapy, that may indicate she's positive and growth-oriented. But if she tells you all about her diagnosis, is obsessed with her therapist, or talks a great deal about her intense emotions, difficult relationships, or childhood traumas, take heed. You're looking for a partner, not a patient.

References to drinking, drugs, or partying can be strong indicators of substance abuse. For the most part, nonabusers aren't talking about drugs or alcohol. Some people deliberately conceal their problems, so this isn't a guarantee—just pay attention and try to get more information. When you do go out with her, notice how much she drinks. Don't let "I must be nervous" be an excuse for three glasses of wine—everyone gets nervous, but drinking to cope isn't a good sign.

➤

Look for signs of good boundaries. Can she talk about herself without spilling her guts too quickly? Do you feel overwhelmed by TMI (too much information)? In the beginning, too much is more problematic than too little. It's good judgment not to share intimate details with strangers—and until you've spent some time interacting face to face, you're still strangers.

Sadly, something that may feel great is also a sign of bad boundaries—like when she says, "We just met, but I feel like I've known you forever." Deep connection? No, more like deep need. Trust takes time to develop. Don't fall into that whirlpool of dysfunction—you'll get sucked in fast.

Notice if she respects your boundaries. Are her questions intrusive? If anything she asks makes you nervous, don't answer. Information is power—don't give it away.

Does she take responsibility for her difficulties? When she talks about a relationship ending, does she say "I wish I'd made better decisions," or "She was a nut"? People who blame others are going to blame you when something goes wrong. Furthermore, they're notoriously resistant to changing, so beware.

You want to find women as sexual as you are, but it's too risky to put that message out right away and online. You don't know each other yet. If she's a nice person, she may be offended, and if she's a predator, you may be in trouble. Also, you can't know if you'll be attracted to someone until you've met her, and vice versa. Sorry: No shortcuts on this one!

Handling Rejection with Grace

Whichever paths we take to find potential partners, we'll reject some, and some will reject us. It's hard to keep our ego intact when someone we don't even know has decided he or she doesn't want us. We have to toughen up our self-image so it doesn't deflate when a first date that seemed full of promise never calls again.

Rejection happens at any age. What makes it harder for us now is that maybe we don't, deep down, feel desirable. That's up to us to change, not up to our dates. Easier said than done, but we've got to try.

ERICA, AGE 64

I'm not thrilled with single life at all. I loved being married. Although my sex life with my ex-husband was unpleasant to nonexistent, I do miss the intimacy of a companion to share my life. I had to put up with a lot of bullshit from my ex-husband, but I still never would have left if he hadn't found someone else.

I've done a lot of Internet dating. It was fun for a while, but then it got stressful and depressing. Too much rejection. I think I'm either too old or too overweight for a lot of men. At my age, I don't feel attractive.

Some older women attract men no matter how old they are. They have the "it" factor. They're not necessarily beautiful, but they radiate self-confidence. My friend's mother had men pursuing her into her eighties. I never had the "it" factor when I was young and pretty, so how am I going to get it now when I really have good reasons not to feel attractive?

I enjoy the freedom of single life, never having to answer to anyone, reading or watching TV until late, having my space to myself. But it is lonely. I seek a gentle, kind, understanding, supportive man. Unfortunately, I wind up being attracted to the same narcissistic types I was attracted to as a young woman.

No, Thank you

Sometimes you'll be the one doing the rejection. I asked sex therapist Isadora Alman for her tips for letting someone down politely:

ADVICE FROM AN EXPERT

Saying No Gracefully

BY ISADORA ALMAN, MFT

I mentioned to a man I knew socially that I would enjoy getting to know him better on a one-to-one basis. He led me over to a quiet corner, took my hand, and looked into my eyes. "You are one of the most . . . (all sorts of lovely adjectives here) women I have ever met. Unfortunately, for me, I seem to have this thing for skinny neurotic blondes. I wish it were different." I felt so special, so appreciated, that it was minutes before I realized that I—a round redhead of fine mental health—had been turned down, and by a master.

Whether it's a request for a date or for sex, you can't say no without hurting the other person's feelings. But you can minimize the damage. If someone pays you the compliment of wanting you, your company, or your body, it's only fair that you return a kindness—not by giving what is asked for if you're not interested, but by making the asker glad she or he took the risk of asking. Here are a few guidelines.

- Self-talk first. Are there are any conditions which, if met, might change your mind, and do you want to put them out there? ("If you weren't already married . . .")

➤

- Position yourself within eye level and touching distance. The blow of bad news can be softened somewhat by a touch on the arm or hand.

- Use "I" speak. Say "I feel" rather than "You make me feel." Include something positive too, such as, "I've enjoyed speaking with you, but ..."

- Say no clearly and unequivocally. No whining, no giggling. If you'd rather kiss a dozen frogs than get together with the one who's asking, then stringing along is not playing fair. You don't need to explain why. "I'm flattered, but no, thank you," is all you need to say.

- Hear the other person out. If a convincing argument is presented, even if seems like a sales pitch, listen politely and then repeat your refusal. If the other person becomes overly insistent, repeat your refusal more firmly.

- Allow the asker his/her dignity. The asker is taking a risk. Acknowledge that, and the other person, by saying something nice that he or she can take away from the encounter along with that awful feeling of rejection.

- Do not say "Let's be friends" or "I'll call you" and not follow through. If you really want a friendship, it's up to you to make the next offer. If your private wish is that this person would disappear from your world, don't imply any future possibilities. It's not honest or nice.

- If the person grabs hold of your body without your consent, all politeness bets are off. "Stop! You are assaulting me!" along with vigorous attempts to leave will cover most such situations.

- Practice. If you find it difficult to say no convincingly, practice in the mirror until your no is believable.

Happy Endings

At sixty-two, Carol Denker met Warren and was astounded by the power of elder love. She dedicated the next years to interviewing and photographing senior couples whose lives had been transformed by love. Their stories became a gorgeous coffee table book celebrating elder love: *Autumn Romance: Stories and Portraits of Love after 50*. Here Denker shares tips from the seniors she interviewed.

ADVICE FROM AN EXPERT

Finding Love after Fifty

BY CAROL DENKER

I asked each couple I interviewed, "What advice would you give someone over fifty who is looking for love?" None of the answers pointed to the best dating site or updating your wardrobe. The responses were almost all about attitude. Our couples recommend you put these practices into place:

➤

1. Love yourself. This was the No. 1 piece of advice from people who have successfully achieved a great relationship later in life. This is a great time to start loving yourself full-out, even if you were not terrific at this in your younger years. "As you love yourself, you can love another," says Pat.

2. Get to really know yourself. You may have spent years trying to please others. Now it's time to get to know yourself in full, delicious detail. Take as much time as you need. "Get to know your deepest values, your deepest thoughts, what you really love," says Nanka, who stopped dating and started journaling. "By the time I met Bob, I knew who I was and could be fully present."

3. Look clearly at the past. Before you jump into another relationship, be complete with the one you've left. "Make peace with yourself about past relationships that didn't work," says Basia. "See your own unworkable patterns and rise above them."

4. Create a life you love. The more positive a life you create for yourself, the more you'll attract positive people into your life. "Create a life that feels right to you, with friends, activities, and places of community that nurture you and foster contentment," says Dorothy. "Be happy, and more happiness will follow."

5. Take a risk; be open to opportunity. Talk to strangers. Be open. "Your soul mate could be standing next to you in line at the market," says Wanda. "Smile and feel positive."

6. Get out there in the world. Dorothy and Rich sang in the same choir. Basia and Ron went to the same talk. Edith and Ray took the same line-dance class, as did Joan and Robert. Bob and Sue met in their Italian class. "Participate in social activities that you love, and you'll meet people with similar passions," says Joan.

7. Be creative and thoughtful when choosing a partner. Look for what you want now. "Don't fall into the belief that the pickings are slim," says Connie. "Picture what you want in a partner and have faith you'll find it."

8. Don't give up. The universe of possibilities is endless! Be patient: Love will come when you least expect it. "You should not think that, because you are older, you don't have the right to feel the beautiful emotion of love," says Manuela. "And while you are waiting, open your heart to life."

TORY, AGE 65

When I began dating again at sixty, after a fallow period, I was wilder, more amused, more adventuresome than ever before, and found few if any impediments to full sexual pleasure. Perhaps orgasm has become less accessible over the age of sixty, but pleasure is fully accessible.

19

Safer Sex — Yes, at Our Age

I'M A PRODUCER at *ABC News Nightline*," the email began. "I'm working on a story about older Americans and sex, specifically HIV/STD prevention. Have you heard from many people who are back in the dating and mating game after divorce or loss of a partner? Do you find that those people are informed about their sexual health?"

"Based on what they tell me," I responded, "I'd say seniors are *informed*, but most don't act on that information."

This email exchange led to my appearance on *ABC News Nightline* as a spokesperson for older-age sex and love, and a commentator on senior sexual health. Part of the program showed me at my computer, reading from the comments I received after publishing the following on my blog:

> *How do you handle sex and dating? You're dating again after years, maybe decades, away from the dating scene. How do you handle sex with a new person? Do you use/ require condoms? What questions do you ask? What steps do you take to protect your sexual health?*

Although I received a couple of responses of "latex every time with everyone," more common were responses in which people admitted to not using protection. I hope that the information in this chapter will help to change that.

Why Aren't We Practicing Safe Sex?

Only one in five sexually active single adults over forty-five reports using a condom regularly, according to "Sex, Romance, and Relationships: AARP Survey of Midlife and Older Adults," a 2009 study of 1,670 adults forty-five and older released in May 2010. Of those survey participants who are single, dating, and having sex, 50 percent of males and 29 percent of females *rarely or never* use protection.[1] We need to change that!

I can understand not wanting to use condoms. It's difficult enough—emotionally and physically—for those of us dating after a later-life divorce or the devastating death of a partner to get involved in sex with a new person, without having to worry about protecting ourselves from STDs. When we experience the exhilaration of lust after a long period of deprivation, the excitement about a partner desiring our aging body, the emotional need for touching and physical contact, who wants to think about condoms?

We came of age before the time of HIV. If we used barrier protection at all, it was so that we wouldn't get pregnant—or, for the boomers, to avoid STDs like herpes, which weren't life-threatening anyway. With fertility behind us, we feel that sex carries few risks. But that's simply not true, as you'll see by the many alarming facts and statistics shown in this chapter.

Unfortunately, the information about ease of STD transmission and the importance of barrier protection is rarely targeted toward our age group. Why? Maybe we're seen as the throwaway generation—old people with one foot in the grave anyway. More likely, it's the ongoing, head-in-the-sand, social attitude that sex among people in our age group is too icky to address, so we're ignored—despite the statistics that have been available from the Centers for Disease Control and Prevention (CDC) for years.

It's not surprising that we're not as aware as we should be of our sexual health risks. Physicians often do not address sexual health with older patients, or discuss our risk for HIV and other STDs. Doctors often don't test older people for HIV, leaving infected patients to transmit the virus to partners without knowing they have it. Even when an older person comes in with early symptoms of HIV—such as fatigue, weakness, and memory changes—doctors may misdiagnose these as normal signs of aging.

I don't want to scare you and have you go running for an HIV test just because you forgot your daughter's phone number or needed a nap yesterday, but I do think it's important to be fully informed. If you've had unprotected sex with someone whose sexual history isn't known to you, please do get tested. It's easy, confidential, and often free of charge or very inexpensive.

Below are some responses I received to my blog post about dating and safer sex. They reflect the real need for sex ed for seniors.

ERICA, AGE 64

I never worried about AIDS or using protection, because I thought it was dumb. I don't know a soul with AIDS or even know anyone who knows anyone with it. What's the chance of my getting it? I figured the men I was sleeping with were, like me, married for the past twenty years, and that they missed out on the AIDS epidemic. I take a lot worse risks every day eating stuff I shouldn't or passing cars on two-lane highways.

SETH, AGE 61

Long gone are the days of easy sex. Now I have lot of conversation beforehand. I got herpes a few years ago from my committed relationship. She never told me, and she had a major breakout while we were together. Since then, in conversations with past relationships, two women admitted that they had herpes and never told me for fear of losing me. Now, if I reconnect with an old mate for a magical evening, I will use a condom.

RACHEL, AGE 62

I came of age sexually during a privileged period. All we had to worry about was pregnancy. No STDs to speak of, and in our milieu, we thought only trashy people got them. I was married for almost twenty years, and when I opened my eyes and looked around, it was a different, scarier world. I'd like to tell you I've been cautious. That'd be a big fat lie. I've never been cautious. Would I recommend my own recklessness to others? Of course not.

KELLY, AGE 70

I have to admit to total ignorance regarding the use of condoms. I cannot truthfully recall ever having been intimate with a condom, and frankly, I have no desire to be now either. They're artificial, and I don't like artifice. Since I'm hardly likely to get pregnant (and that was their primary function), I thought I'd never need to hear about them again. But then came AIDS. So how does one handle that situation?

EVELYNN, AGE 65

I don't think of sexual encounters as dangerous unless I *feel* that there is a threat of danger. I protect myself by not engaging in sexual activities with a new partner until I am sure that we are meeting on the same vibrational level.

ANNA, AGE 64

I recently taught a sexuality class at my church, and I warned the kids that they must use condoms. But when it came to my having sex, I did nothing past asking new partners if they had any diseases. None of the men insisted on wearing them either, after I reassured them that I am healthy. I depend on a person's intelligence, experience, past lifestyle, and facts about their life to piece together a confidence that he is being truthful with me when he says he has no diseases. I have been on a bit of a sexual tear the last few years and have had many partners. When I tell my prospective partners this, instead of turning away from me as a health risk, it seems to turn them on.

GERARD, AGE 63

I've been in the "dating after being married a long time" world for eight years. During that time, I've had twenty-five sexual partners. Most of the women were from a similar background as me—professional, well-educated, previously married. We came of sexual age when sex was free and easy and perceived as almost an entitlement.

Of those twenty-five sexual partners I've had as a geezer, only one insisted on me using a condom. And she was one I met in a swingers' environment, where she was having lots of partners. Maybe three others initially brought up a half-hearted request after things were getting libidinous: "Uh, you're going to use a condom, aren't you? *pant pant*" A reply of "I haven't had many partners lately *pant pant*" put it to rest. And as for the other twenty-one partners, the topic of condoms never came up.

TORY, AGE 65

I've dated men I met on the Internet and enjoyed multiple partners in a sex club. I just gauge the partner before having sex with him. If it's in a sex club or someplace anonymous, I insist on a condom. Otherwise, I don't protect myself, except by querying the partner before having sex as to whether he has any diseases. I listen to his answer and take his word for it. I generally trust my reaction to the person.

HIV at Our Age

Sexually transmitted infections, particularly HIV/AIDS, are increasing in the fifty-plus age group. In the United States, the CDC reported in 2005 that adults age fifty and older accounted for the following.

- 15 percent of new HIV/AIDS diagnoses

- 24 percent of persons living with HIV/AIDS (increased from 17 percent in 2001)

- 19 percent of all AIDS diagnoses

- 29 percent of persons living with AIDS

- 35 percent of all deaths of persons with AIDS

The CDC also estimates that by 2015, half of the one million Americans living with HIV will be older than fifty.[2]

Those facts about HIV/AIDS among older adults may be surprising. But that's not all. Take a look at these facts, which I hope will make you nervous about having unsafe sex.

- According to the National Institute on Aging, older people often mistake signs of HIV/AIDS as normal age-related aches and pains, and often have the virus for years without being aware they are infected.[3]

- A University of Chicago study found that nearly 60 percent of unmarried women ages fifty-eight to ninety-three who had been sexually active in the previous ten years reported that they had not used a condom.[4]

- About half of the older people with AIDS have been infected for one year or less.[5]

- An Ohio University study found that about 27 percent of HIV-infected men and 35 percent of HIV-infected women over fifty sometimes have sex without using condoms.[6]

- According to the CDC, older women are particularly at risk for blood-borne diseases like HIV or chlamydia because their thinning vaginal lining and lack of lubrication lead to vaginal-wall tearing during intercourse, permitting easy access to the bloodstream.[7]

Safer-Sex Role Models

I found it interesting that of the people who responded to my safer-sex question, the ones who were having the most sex with the most partners were often also the ones who never had unprotected sex.

TINGGI, AGE 61

I wish society and the media would treat sex as expected, normal activity at any age—sort of like eating and sleeping. I like to indulge in erotic activity daily with myself or others, and I have intercourse with one to three partners a week. I consider myself bisexual. I tend to have several partners at the same time. All of the relationships are open, and all my partners regularly have sex with others. I'm diligent about practicing safer sex, and I have not had partner sex without a condom in more than thirty years.

My barrier policy is standard, long-fixed, and known by all who have shared erotic times with me: Barriers are always used—for everyone, every time—for any genital contact. This "every time, everyone" policy makes life simpler—no need for elaborate calculations as to number of partners, who they were, days since last STD check-up, partners since our last date, etc. When sex is likely—or probable, or possible, or even a wisp of my imagination—I bring my own supply of barriers. Should the opportunity arise, when we have both shed our clothes, I simply say, "Okay, now it's time to get Charles (not *my* name) dressed," and I put on a condom.

When dates insist on sex without a condom (which rarely happens), the date becomes a chaste one and a last one. Steady dates (people with whom I have sex repeatedly) get the same treatment each date: "every time, everyone." I have had dates thank me for using a barrier, and for being a guy they can trust to always use one. A successful line is "I'm not worried about catching something from you, I'm sure you are quite healthy. I'm worried about giving something to you."

I have myself checked for STDs some four times a year at a clinic specializing in such. No STD has been detected in the over three decades of the "every time, everyone" policy. Such was *not* the case prior to my adoption of this policy.

I don't ask dates about their sexual history, because I am going to use barriers regardless. People can have an STD and show no detectable signs outside of a laboratory test.

Barrier use can be eroticized to become a fun and arousing part of sexual interaction. I believe this "every time, everyone" policy protects my dates, myself, and my community. A sad fact is that HIV is being transmitted in our retirement homes by the residents. It is already there, waiting for me.

PAMM, AGE 54

I'm not interested in playing with others who don't care enough about themselves to practice safer sex. I have swinging experience. At swingers' events, you put condoms out all over the place—just as you do mints! You make agreements beforehand to be conscious and responsible.

Not only do you use condoms, but you *have* to change them in between partners. You should be washing your hands with sanitizer in between partners too.

In my experience and beliefs, conscious, safety-minded people can easily take a minute to be safe. Although my swinging days are over (done there, been that), I would have left the party if condoms weren't being used. That would be irresponsible.

But if you're not leading a life as sexually adventuresome as Tinggi's or Pamm's, and you just want to be sure you're safe before you get into an exclusive relationship with a new person, Paul's or Nina's solution might be just right for you.

PAUL, AGE 51

I always request a blood test prior to a new relationship. I go to my county clinic or Planned Parenthood, where the testing is free. The results take a week or so. For me, it's clearly preferable to the stretch-and-snap, hair-catching, smells-like-glue condom. I've slept with four women in the six years since my divorce, and in each case, we got the blood test. I bring it up when the prospect of sex seems good, after three or four weeks.

NINA, AGE 67

My partners and I always use condoms for intercourse until, and only if, we decide that we will be primary, monogamous partners for the foreseeable future. Then we get tested and show each other our results before ceasing condom use. If the test results are negative, and only then, we can go condomless. Even if his history is, say, that he's only had one partner in the past five years, and that he and she were tested before having unprotected intercourse—and even if I trust him to be telling me the truth—we will use condoms until our tests come back negative.

Condom Conversation

Never wait until the heat of passion to bring up the subject. Instead, when the sparks and kisses signal that sex is likely in your future, have The Discussion. Agree to be prepared when you're ready for the next stage, whether that means next weekend, weeks from now, or in an hour.

In my single past, these approaches served me well:

- "I always use condoms with a new partner, to protect us both."

- "I'll buy the condoms—do you prefer a special kind?"

- "Do you have condoms, or should we make a run to the store?"

- "Your condoms or mine?"

- "How many of these do you think we'll need tonight?" (Thanks, with fond memories, to the man who uttered this to me, pointing out his stash of several dozen condoms.)

When Robert and I first became sexual, we got blood tests and used condoms through the waiting time. He had been celibate for four years. I had been much more sexually active in the past years. At the time I met him, I was involved in what today's generation calls a "friends with benefits" relationship with a dear, longtime pal. I knew my friend's sexual history, and he and I had been tested before deciding we could forego condoms. But Robert was understandably uneasy about what I might be bringing to the relationship, and I was happy to use condoms for his peace of mind until our test results proclaimed us both "safe."

I talked to Robert about how difficult it is for many dating singles of our age to talk about safer sex. "In any deepening of a relationship, sharing beliefs in an honest manner is a way of bonding," he told me. "While I don't like condoms, I believe in using them until we've been tested, and waiting out that period. This demonstrates that you care for the other person and yourself."

I told him that some women are shy about having condoms ready, worrying their partners might think less of them. "If a woman already has the condoms on hand, I think, *That's a smart woman*," Robert said. "Whoever is hosting the interlude should have condoms. That makes a good impression, like having coffee and milk on hand in case he stays over."

ADVICE FROM AN EXPERT

Safer Sex 101 for Seniors

BY MICHELE CAUCH, MA, MSW

Age is not a barrier against sexually transmitted infections (STIs)—in fact, older women are more at risk, because the vaginal lining is thinner due to lowered estrogen. It is up to you to make an informed decision about your body and sexuality. Here are your safer-sex basics.

Condoms: Those Circular Impressions in Your Wallet

Aside from abstinence, condoms are the most effective method to protect against sexually transmitted infections.

- Explore condom options. Condoms come in a variety of styles: ribbed, studded, spiral, twisted, flared, baggy, multitextured, colored, glow-in-the-dark, lubricated, and different sizes. There are also female condoms, which allow women to take more control over their sexual health. Visit your local sex shop and get to know what's out there. You'll be amazed at the selection. If your partner feels uncomfortable buying condoms, take the initiative and buy them yourself.

- Take responsibility. Carry condoms with you if there's any chance you'll be sexually active. Never assume your partner has or will use condoms.

- Be creative and spice things up by making condoms a part of your foreplay. It can be very sexy when a partner puts the condom on the man. Let your partner know that a positive approach to safe sex is a turn-on.

➤

➤

- Choose latex or polyurethane condoms. Polyurethane is recommended, as some people can have an allergic reaction to latex.

- Never re-use a condom. It is unhygienic and dangerous. Latex and polyurethane are thin, fragile materials, which can tear during intercourse. Infected body fluids can pass through microscopic holes.

Communicating with Your Partner

Educate yourself first on the "why" and the "how" of safer-sex practices so that you can talk with a new partner before you become intimate. Learning about safer sex will increase your comfort level and help to demystify the subject.

Talking about sexuality is what most of us learned not to do, but it's never too late to develop the skill of communicating effectively and directly. Find out how a new partner feels about condoms, and express your concerns about safe sex. Initiate discussion before you get to the bedroom. Older adults need to begin talking about this subject, so that others will learn about protecting themselves.

Discuss your commitment to protecting the sexual health of both of you. Use "I" statements, such as the following:

- "I've heard there are condoms that increase pleasure for women. Let's try them."

- "I'm really turned on by you, and I want to have safe sex to protect both of us."

If your partner refuses to practice safer sex or is unsympathetic to your concerns, is this partner right for you? You are ultimately responsible for your sexual health.

Female Condoms

If you're a woman whose male partner can't use a regular condom—or if you, the woman, want to be in charge of making sure you're covered, so to speak—try a female condom. These odd-looking contraptions fit inside the vagina and protrude, with rings to hold them in place. If you tried a female condom decades ago, as I did, you remember that it sounded and felt like making love in a shower curtain. The new model, FC2, is greatly improved. Here's how the official FC2 website, www.fc2.us.com, describes the female condom:

> FC2 Female Condom is a thin, soft, loose-fitting sheath made from synthetic rubber (nonlatex), which is worn inside the vagina. There is a flexible ring at each end. The inner ring, at the closed end of the sheath, is used to insert the condom inside the vagina and to hold it in place during intercourse. The rolled outer ring, at the open end of the sheath, remains outside the vagina and covers part of the external genitalia.

Female condoms are more expensive than regular condoms but have great advantages. The woman inserts it herself, so it doesn't affect or require the man's erection. Men say that the sensation is better than with a male condom. More spontaneity is possible, because it can be inserted in advance, and it doesn't have to be removed immediately after ejaculation.

Eroticizing Condoms

"It's hard enough to get guys my age hard in the first place, much less stopping to put on a rubber."
    ERICA, AGE 64

Many men of our age have enough difficulty getting and maintaining erections without having to put another barrier—literally—between an unreliable penis and a welcoming partner. Even young men frequently lose erections when they stop to put on a condom.

The solution isn't to toss the condoms in the trash but to find ways to eroticize condom use. I always found the moment very erotic when my partner reached for a condom—it meant he knew I was ready for him. The sound of the condom package ripping open was a turn-on—he would soon be inside me.

Make condom use an erotic part of sex play. Keep them on the bedside table in an elegant box or basket that you can easily reach, rather than hiding them away in a drawer. Make sure all the discussions about safer sex have already taken place, so it's understood that one of you will reach for the condom when the time comes. If he enjoys it, use a vibrator to give his penis a boost before or after dressing him with a condom. Keep the foreplay going—keep kissing and stroking while the condom is going on, and afterward.

Advice to Older Men about Condoms

CHARLIE GLICKMAN, PHD

Older men and their partners tell me that erection difficulties are a barrier to condom use. It seems to be a combination of the effect of anxiety on erection and, for some men, the act of putting on the condom, which may squeeze blood out of the penis.

For anxiety, I recommend practicing with a condom during solo sex for a while, to help build the skills. If you're more confident at putting condoms on and can do it more quickly, it's less likely to cause problems. Mostly, it's a matter of practice.

When you're with a partner, keep the supplies near the bed so you don't have to hunt for them. You can open the condom in advance and set it aside until you need it.

Make sure that your partner is ready for intercourse before you put it on. Keep up the level of sexual energy—through kissing, oral sex, fantasy talk, and whatever else works for you—to keep safer sex from interrupting things.

To keep from squeezing blood out of the penis while putting on the condom, it helps a lot to do your PC-muscle exercises. This is the muscle that contracts and releases during orgasm. In men, it makes the penis bounce and the anus grip, and it helps propel ejaculate.

Learn how to contract the PC muscle voluntarily by stopping the flow of urine. It's best to sit on the toilet while doing this (if you stand, you risk making a mess) or to practice in the shower. Then, once you've found this muscle, work it out by

➤

> clenching and releasing, trying different rhythms. You can do
this while masturbating or in completely nonsexual settings.

Many men report that their erections get firmer with
PC-muscle exercises, because the muscle helps keep blood in
the penis. If the pressure from rolling a condom on is greater
that the PC-muscle's ability to do that, you're basically squeezing the blood out, similar to squeezing a tube of toothpaste.
What a metaphor!

Some men have found that cock rings can help them maintain an erection during condom use, although I think a strong
PC muscle is a better choice—unless you enjoy the way the
cock rings feel. Cock rings are worn around the shaft of the
penis, usually behind the scrotum—although some men prefer
to wear them in front of the testicles. Blood flows in through
the center of the penis and back out closer to the surface.
Wearing a cock ring around the base of the penis restricts the
blood flow and creates a sensation of tightness and pressure
that many men enjoy.

No Excuses

Many of you have told me that you ask potential partners about
their sexual health and history and accept their answers. I hate to
be the one to tell you, but people lie about their pasts and their
risks—especially if they're panting to touch you naked. Often
they don't even know whether they have a sexually transmitted
infection.

You trust your intuition? Personally, I've been duped by my
intuition, in bed and out. I hired a contractor who charmed me,
conned me, and cost me thousands of dollars. I loved a man for

eight years who lied and cheated on me, and I had no clue at the time. And, like many women, I've had my share of men who wooed me, bedded me, and never called again. I've learned from my mistakes not to take chances with my sexual health.

"Don't you trust me?" your partner may ask if you insist on a condom. Trust is beside the point. Many people have sexually transmitted infections without knowing it—not just HIV, but herpes, chlamydia, and more. For example, some people who know they have herpes (which is treatable but not curable) may decide that they don't need to reveal this if their herpes is not active.

Some of my women readers write me that they feel uncomfortable asking a new partner to use a condom. They are newly in the dating game after divorce or death of a partner. "If I ask a man to use a condom, it sounds like I don't trust him," they say. "If I have them on hand myself, he'll think I sleep around."

My belief is that if you can't talk about safer sex with someone, do you really want to invite that person inside your body? I know it's hard, especially if you've been in a long-term relationship and suddenly find yourself out in that scary world of dating, sex with new partners, and risks that weren't a part of our blazing youth.

I don't claim that I used a condom with everyone all the time when I was single. In my younger days, the STDs we were likely to contact were either visible or could be cured with a prescription drug. But I got smarter with age and became more demanding of barrier protection. If I knew someone well already—someone who had become a good friend, and I knew about his relationships and his sexual health status—we would get blood tests, and then feel comfortable about condomless sex. But that took deep discussions and friendship.

I know it's embarrassing to insist on more than a verbal assurance, but it's essential these days. If someone is offended that you won't have unprotected sex, please get your clothes back on. Potential partners who are this casual with your sexual health and their own have done this before, you can bet—and do you really want to sleep with all the people he or she has slept with, and all of those people's casual partners?

I've had occasions when a man refused to use a condom, saying something like, "Sex with condoms just isn't enjoyable."

I would reply, "Is *no* sex more enjoyable?"

At this point, I knew the date was over, and I was glad to know in advance that he didn't value my sexual health or his own. If he was willing to go to bed with me without protection, then he did that with his last partners, and they did it with their last partners, and so on.

The message is this: If you're dating and sexually active, please use condoms, whatever your age, until and unless you're in an exclusive relationship and have both tested negative for sexually transmitted infections. Men complain to me that condoms make sex less pleasurable, and women insist that they're not at risk and are embarrassed to insist on condoms. Haven't we heard variations on these objections from youth? Isn't this one area where we can learn from experience and our own good sense?

20

Better Now Than Ever:
The Joys of Older-Age Sex

B *etter Than I Ever Expected: Straight Talk about Sex after Sixty* celebrated the joys of senior sex, and *Naked at Our Age* aims to help if you are not having great sex. Despite all the problems you wrote me about since *Better Than I Ever Expected* was published, many of you continue to describe relationships that are, indeed, better than you ever expected. When the love, passion, communication, and connection are present, it almost doesn't matter whether erections are strong or orgasms come easily.

When sex is no longer a biological imperative—when we're not driven by our hormones—arousal and satisfaction feel different. Not better, not worse, but different. We make love more spiritually, perhaps, or more slowly, or both. We love kissing and touching, and sometimes don't care whether these lead to intercourse. When our bodies join physically, we may feel that the *emotional* bonding surpasses orgasm in importance and satisfaction. That doesn't mean we've stopped having or wanting orgasms—we do love our orgasms. But sexuality is more than that, and often without goals.

This chapter showcases your comments illustrating that great sex—and love and intimacy—are attainable at our age. We find exhilaration and passion with our partner, or on our own, and we're amazed at how fulfilling our sexuality can be in our later years. Who knew? Certainly no one told us to expect it!

New Lovers, Great Sex

Raquel and Milo are in the heady stage of new love. They each describe how turned on they are to each other.

RAQUEL, AGE 53

Milo and I have been together eleven months. Sex is far better than I ever imagined it could be. Here I am, madly in love with a wonderful man who is passionate about pleasuring me. For the first time in my life, I am completely uninhibited. I regularly have multiple orgasms, sometimes up to seven in one session. I cannot imagine being more sexually satisfied. I've never been in a relationship that enabled me to be so open and trusting.

As we have gotten to know each other, we both get aroused more easily. I love how he makes love to my breasts. I love how he goes down on me. I love when he reaches for the "toy box" while we are making love, and watches me get myself off with a vibrator, then thrusts himself inside me to come. I could go on and on about how this man turns me on!

MILO, AGE 58

It is really hot that Raquel knows how to get herself off. She is a sexual tigress—comfortable with herself, confident in her actions, and willing to share her sexual desires. When I was younger, the thought of sex was enough to turn me on. It was all about "me" rather than about "us." Now what really turns me on is seeing my partner turned on, which comes from her sexual maturity and self-knowledge.

In the beginning of our relationship, I experienced what I thought was erectile dysfunction. My doctor suggested that it might be more psychological than medical in nature, because I'm extremely healthy. At my request, he prescribed Cialis, which we used with mixed results.

In hindsight, my erection issue was more about my psyche than a medical condition. We became more closely connected and stopped using the medications. Erections come slower than when I was younger, but in no way does it diminish our pleasure. We have a splendid sexual relationship.

As a child, my parents never spoke about sexuality and expected me not to act on it. As a young adult, I felt guilty about having sexual desires. I thought that sex was for procreation rather than for pleasure, so I didn't even feel right about having sex with my wife. A pattern of failed marriages and relationships followed—in large part due to lack of the intimacy that comes from a healthy sexual relationship. I finally sought counseling. That was one of the best things I've done, as it opened my eyes to the possibilities sexual intimacy can bring to a relationship.

Sex, Plus Wisdom and Experience

These wonderful stories make me marvel at how much more able we are to truly enjoy sex at our age than we were in our youth.

MIRIAM, AGE 57

I love the casual pace of making love for three hours: the caressing, gazing, and excruciatingly arousing touch before and during orgasm. The older we get, the more of ourselves there is to give, back and forth, in those fabulous lovemaking sessions. There's nothing to prove, just love given, back and forth.

I'm way more sexually mature, loving, skilled, adventurous, and appreciative at this age than in my earlier decades. If only the younger generation knew this, so they could look forward to these fabulous sexual years in old age! Wouldn't that turn our culture's expectations for sexual happiness and contentment inside out?

RALPH, AGE 75

When I was younger, I observed teenaged couples walking home from school. The boy would have his arm over the girl's shoulder, letting his hand drape over her breast. I'm sure that he was telling her how much he loved her, and what a bright future they were going to have together. The truth is that he wanted to find a vagina for his hard-on, plain and simple.

Older-age sexuality comes with maturity and understanding. Sex at our age is expressive, not rushed, and certainly not taken for granted. Just think how many social problems would be prevented if the urge and potential got stronger as we grew older and was less strong for the young. We understand those precious times of loving, giving, sharing, and feeling. We are careful and considerate and let our mate understand how special she is. We take time to appreciate the art of lovemaking.

ED, AGE 52

The best thing about sex is the package of what it has become with my spouse. I love its frequency, dynamic, expression, and feeling. I like that it has become the expression of our love. When we were young, we didn't know much beyond the basics, and together we learned sexual skills over time. At our age, we are more open to new experiences. We feel free to speak about the pleasures we would like to experience. We have memories that we treasure and that make my heart race.

Sex in our twenties was quick and simple. Sometimes all she had to do was touch me, and bam, my ejaculation was over. During my late twenties, my ejaculations began to stop flying across my wife's back and instead simply spurt out. My endurance began to grow during my thirties, and sex might go all night. Sex was more desirable than sleep.

During my forties, my erections began to soften a little. I don't think that this has been any detriment, because it allows for more sex play in a variety of ways. During my younger years, we could never enjoy multiple positions and games for long before an ejaculation. Now we can.

Sex now in my oncoming golden years rubs my soul. I enjoy all of it. My wife turns me on: her attitude, her way of preparing for sex, her hot body, her way of touching, her willingness to experiment, her scent and feel, her softness and gentle way.

The basic difference is that sex in our young days involved an erect and hard penis that was instantaneously ready to ejaculate and mostly did with little notice. But now there is time for play and sexual adventures in bed well before the erection begins.

EVE, AGE 61

Sex is more meaningful and pleasurable, even with all the physical problems of aging. There is a joyfulness and spiritual quality to our lovemaking that was never there when I was younger. I have many illnesses, and as I age they just get worse, but God gave me the *best* man I have ever known to love me. I constantly say, "God saved the best for last." My husband's erectile difficulties give me a chance to initiate the activity and bring him to an erection by stimulating him in a number of ways. It makes me feel sensual and sexy that I am able to affect him in such a wonderful way! I see his desire in his eyes and in the love and attention he gives me every hour of my day. And he has the most beautiful penis I have ever seen.

BEN, AGE 69

I am slower to have an erection, but then the enjoyment is even greater than before. We enjoy sex more now than at any time in our lives. We both work at keeping sex exciting and enjoyable. My wife gives me oral sex until I have an erection, or I enter her while soft and get an erection afterward. Some positions make it possible to enter without an erection. We hug, and I play with her breasts until I have an erection. Many times I have an orgasm without ejaculating. Sometimes we will make love for hours, and my wife will have several orgasms. Our sex is the best my wife and I have ever enjoyed. There is no rushing to orgasm. Just go slow and enjoy the pleasure.

CHLOE, AGE 70

I love the ability to have sex at anytime without interruption, take as long as we want, be as loud as we want, and do it anywhere we want. It is freedom, in every way possible. When we had children at home, we were never able to yell out, talk dirty, and moan when we were having sex. Now anything goes.

OLIVIA, AGE 69

Old people hold hands more and have learned the wisdom of how to comfort each other and to be honest about what they want, because they are running out of time to fulfill themselves. There is a promise of joy that can sustain us through the losses and crises of bodies losing their ability to replenish dying cells. If you nurture sex, it won't desert you. Some change is inevitable, but you don't have to lose it all, ever.

JORDANA, AGE 55

My orgasms are much more powerful than they were in my youth. I don't think I actually understood *how* to have an orgasm when I was younger. I certainly got more aroused back then, but it was more of a fever pitch, and less of a deep orgasm, which is now part of my sexual experiences with my husband of almost twenty years.

CHRISTINE, AGE 49

I know what makes me happy and turned on. I am more comfortable talking about sex—before, during, and after. I understand men a lot better now, and that makes me a better lover. My sexuality oozes out of everything that I am. I love trying new things, and not being all hung up if they don't work. We tease each other sexually throughout the day, verbally and through texts and emails. The anticipation is sometimes half the fun. By the time we get in bed, we want to tear each other's clothes off.

VITALI, AGE 70

My partner had hip-replacement surgery and experienced less sexual desire, resulting in a reduction of sexual frequency. I adapted willingly and noticed that, contrary to my expectations, my sexual satisfaction was not diminished. If anything, it got better. I'm astonished by the degree of sexual satisfaction I've enjoyed with my partner over the past twenty-two years. Our sexual relationship is as satisfying to me now as it was when we met.

SCRUFFY, AGE 57

I am a sexual being capable of giving and receiving pleasure from both genders. When I was first exploring my sexuality,

I felt like I was the only person in the whole wide world with the feelings I had. I was attracted to other boys and didn't even have a name for what I felt. It was a lonely, scary time for me.

In my younger days, sex was just notches on the bedpost. It's about quality nowadays. The pressure is off—I don't have to prove anything. I've also managed to acquire a well-rounded sexual skill set through the years.

I have a fairly active sex life that currently includes one female partner in addition to my self-pleasuring practices. I'm willing to experiment and don't limit myself to penis/vagina sex. Penetrative sex doesn't have to be the Holy Grail of sexual activity. We're only limited by our preconceived notions and our imagination. I've had hours-long sessions with a partner where we just touched and/or massaged each other's bodies, occasionally venturing to the "nether regions" with nothing more than a light touch. The experience was amazing!

I've been HIV-positive for twenty years and figured I would be pretty much left to my own devices. So I relearned how to pleasure myself. Toys and various masturbatory devices opened up a whole different set of sensations. When I am with a partner, everything I've learned about my body and its responses while self-pleasuring translates to partnered sex.

I disclose my HIV-positive status to my partners from the beginning. I use safe sex practices *always*. If a normally healthy individual gets an STI, it's certainly not a good thing. But for someone with an already compromised immune system, the consequences could be devastating.

I'm pretty much fully functional, with occasional erectile difficulties. But hey, that's what tongues and fingers are for. My erectile difficulties can be frustrating, but even without an erection, I enjoy touch, talk, fantasy, and massage. I have a rich sex life, thanks to my experience, openness, sense of humor, and ability to communicate.

If we believe that being sexual ends with a number, then that's our fate. If instead we embrace the changes and challenges, and acknowledge our bodies as they are instead of pining for what they once were, then we can have a rich and rewarding sex life for as long as we live.

BESS, AGE 67

We touch each other as if in foreplay when we are out in public, dancing. We get away with it, because we are this "cute old couple who are obviously in love." In the evenings, I'll put on music and dance for him, seducing him to join me. I rub my body against his in sexy ways. Eventually we wind up making love. I take a lot of the responsibility for keeping things sexy, and I know he appreciates it—I think he rides a lot on my sexual energy.

KAT, AGE 51

Sex at fifty-plus is way better than it was in my twenties for many great reasons. Don't think we aren't thinking sexy thoughts, having incredible fantasies (maybe about you, laddie, behind the counter at Starbucks), and even sometimes acting on those fantasies. We're over fifty, we're sexy, and we're proud, and we're not afraid to say it out loud!

Nurturing Intimacy in Long-Term Relationships

Many couples write me that the sex has gone out of a loving relationship, with comfortable familiarity replacing the dizzy, exhilarating sex of courtship. The "bonding" brain chemicals replace the high-powered "lust and attraction" brain chemicals, and that "Gotta touch you now!" drive becomes "Let's just cuddle."

The thing is, couples who keep their sexual relationship strong also experience powerful, emotional bonding (especially at our age), while those who let the lust go often find the emotional intimacy drifting away as well. When our hormones stop driving our sex lives, we need to be intentional about sex, to nurture it and make it happen. We're capable of great, glorious orgasms our whole lives, but we have to make a point of creating space in our calendars and in our emotions for them to happen.

This section offers some excellent advice from experts on how to keep love, sex, and intimacy alive, no matter how long you've been with your partner.

ADVICE FROM AN EXPERT

24-Hour Foreplay:
The Secret of Long-Term Lovers

GLENDA CORWIN, PHD

The unfortunate reality is that a majority of couples, after the early romantic phase of their relationship, drift into a pattern of having sex rarely, or never. But not all. Long-term, sexually active couples have a secret: They are intentional about their sexual relationship. They set aside time for intimacy and engage in sensual activities and erotic imagination to get in the mood. They consciously and deliberately practice what I call "24-hour foreplay."

By foreplay, I mean the activities that you do *before* a potential sexual encounter. Do you remember how spontaneous

➤

sexual desire felt when you first started dating someone? Actually, it wasn't spontaneous at all—you created most of it by careful planning and anticipation. How did you get ready for a sexy date? Did you arrange to be uninterrupted? Did you wear something sensual? Did you imagine how it would feel to embrace, or did you visualize sexual scenes? Did you do any of this even the day *before* your date? *That's* 24-hour foreplay.

24-hour foreplay includes:

- Sensual awareness: Spend time making your body feel good, such as a hot bath or stretching.

- Erotic imagination: Let sexual fantasies turn you on.

- Emotional connection: Bond with sweet-talking phone calls or emails.

All this happens long before your actual date.

Beware of the Self-Sabotage Demon. You know exactly how to screw up a sexual opportunity. Start an argument. Make a phone call. Start on a household project. All of these can completely destroy sexual energy. Avoid distractions and just focus on your love date. Every time you make plans to make love, you're validating your sexuality, and that's good for both of you.

Tips for Romancing Your Partner

BY TINA B. TESSINA, PHD

Whether your relationship is new or decades old, keep letting your partner know how much you love him or her, both verbally and through actions. Here are some ways:

- Touch each other. Touch as often as possible, not just when you want sex. Sit close and gently place your hand on your partner's shoulder, leg, or arm. Your conversation will become warmer and more caring, opening the way to sexual expression.

- Change stress to silliness. Laugh frequently, especially if things are frustrating. Ease the tension with light humor. Don't poke fun at your mate, but use shared humor as a way to say, "I know this is tough, but we'll get through it." Shared laughter sets the stage for shared intimacy.

- Surprise your partner. Leave a love note in your partner's briefcase; give a flower or card for no reason. An unexpected hug or kiss says, "I'm thinking good thoughts about you, and I love you." Partners who feel loved during the day want to be closer at night.

- Ramp up the sweetness. Married life has its unavoidable stresses. Add a spritz of sweetness frequently. Thank-yous and gestures of politeness and affection are the WD-40 of your marriage, especially when

➤

things are strained. Be the main source of sweetness for each other.

- Celebrate and appreciate each other. No matter how crazed you are with work, health concerns, or bills, put aside regular time each week for a date night. Keep connected, don't let stress build up, and affirm how good you are together.

- Reminisce about good times. "Remember when . . ." is a great start to a loving conversation. Reminisce about when you were dating, when you got married, when you had your first child, when your child left the nest. Reminding yourselves of your solid history together increases your bond.

- Brag to friends. Tell your mate how much you care privately, but also tell your friends and family, while your mate is around, what a great guy or gal you're with, such as, "He really understands me," or "I'm so lucky to be in this relationship." Despite embarrassment, your partner will be pleased and remember what you said. And what's more fun than sex with your biggest fan?

Advice for Good Sex

BY DR. DAVID HERSH

Hide all clocks in the room. Shut all telephone ringers. There are no goals in bed. The whole body is potentially erotic. Keep your eyes open. Talk to your partner during sex. Laugh. Yes, you really can have sex for eight hours. Sex is not necessarily about intercourse or orgasm. It's about scratching the itch, and occasionally, one can reach transcendence.

Plan ahead. When you're going to have sex, set up your space with anything you might need—towels, lots of lube, refreshments, music, videos—so you don't have to jump up and break the mood. If sex is not happening spontaneously for you, plan for sex. Then spontaneity may return.

Sex is about having fun. Own your sexuality. Ask for sex. Initiate it. Claim your power.

ADVICE FROM AN EXPERT

Bonding with a Daily Snuggle

MARNIA ROBINSON

"Bonding behaviors" are subconscious signals that can make emotional ties surprisingly effortless. Try these bonding behaviors to revive and strengthen the closeness in your relationship:

- smiling, with eye contact

➤

- skin-to-skin contact

- unsolicited approval, via smiles or compliments

- gazing into each other's eyes

- synchronized breathing

- kissing with lips and tongues

- holding or spooning each other in stillness

- wordless sounds of contentment and pleasure

- providing a service or treat without being asked

- offering comfort through stroking or hugging

- placing your palm gently over your lover's genitals with intent to comfort, not arouse

- making time together at bedtime a priority

Nurture the closeness in your relationship daily with these bonding behaviors. Make them genuinely selfless. The more you use bonding behaviors, the more sensitive your brain becomes to the neurochemicals that help you feel relaxed and loving. Even holding each other in stillness at the end of a busy day can be enough to exchange the subconscious signals that your relationship is rewarding.

Some of these behaviors may sound like foreplay, but that's not their intent. Foreplay is aimed at building sexual tension and climax. Bonding behaviors are aimed at relaxation and peaceful connection. Bonding behaviors can restore and sustain the harmonious sparkle in a relationship with surprising ease.

In Robert's Words

My beloved Robert died at age seventy-one. Almost right up to the end of his life, Robert actively supported my dream of this book, knowing he would not live to read it. During the last weeks that we were able to walk in the park together, we discussed this book—what would be in it, how it would expand on topics brought up in *Better Than I Ever Expected*, and what new topics it would need.

I hadn't yet come up with a good title, and Robert left me little penciled notes with ideas on used envelopes and sales receipts. (He never started a new piece of paper when an old one would do.) We brainstormed together incessantly.

I would read him emails and excerpts from interviews that were coming in, and he would listen compassionately to the concerns readers wrote me. Sometimes he would sit down in my study and start talking, and I would scramble to type what he said.

That's what happened here, one year before Robert died. At the time, his leukemia and lymphoma were in remission, and although he felt beaten down by six months of chemo, his vigor, creativity, and sexuality were strong and central to his feelings of well-being. Robert embraced being an elder and felt compelled to share what he had learned. I am grateful to him for this, as well as for everything else he gave me and others.

"Sexuality as I Have Experienced It"

BY ROBERT RICE

When asked what is most important about sexuality as I have experienced it, here is what I say:

- Some form of sexual expression is essential for optimal health and happiness.
- Feeling sexy is our own responsibility. Waiting to be turned on is arrogant.
- Orgasm is a human experience in synchrony with the pulse of nature and the rhythm of the universe. It takes place outside boundaries of time.
- Some people wear their sexuality with such comfort they radiate sexual energy even when working a crossword puzzle.
- When the body seems to have abandoned sexuality, it may be an illusion.
- Sexuality is fluid. There are times throughout life when sex feels urgently needed and other times when the desire is weak or seemingly nonexistent. The length of time that one or the other exists may vary greatly and is conditioned by other life events or by reasons unknown.
- Play and creativity are the two most important ingredients in sexual expression.
- The penis and clitoris are but two of many sensitive body parts.
- We elders who have lived a long, sexually active life are among the best resources on sexuality for younger people, because what we have to teach is tempered by wisdom more than libido.

Put Your Head on My Shoulder

One day I was rushing about, I don't remember for what, maybe preparing for a trip. I was stressed, crashing about, full of nervous energy. Robert caught me in midflight, taking my hand. "I'm so busy," I protested.

"Just for a minute," he said quietly, leading me into the living room.

He switched on the CD player, and Michael Bublé began to sing, *Put Your Head on My Shoulder*. Robert enveloped me in his arms and began to dance me around the room. My body melted into his strong embrace and his graceful rhythm. I started to cry, feeling his closeness and knowing that nothing was more important than holding this man I loved in my arms. I continued to sob, and he didn't need to ask why. He just cradled my head into his shoulder and kept us dancing.

I don't remember what I was rushing to that day, but I do remember every moment in Robert's arms, the feel of his chest against my face, and his body leading mine until our rhythms melted into one being. Yes, just like making love.

I would do anything to dance in his arms again. I narrate this special moment to remind you to stop, take time with your lover if you're fortunate enough to have him or her with you, and never take for granted that there will always be time later on. There won't. Now is all we have. Love each other passionately and tenderly. Treasure each other.

That, in the end, is all that truly matters.

MEET OUR EXPERTS

You can find this list with hyperlinks at
www.NakedAtOurAge.com.

ISADORA ALMAN, MFT, is a board-certified sexologist, a California-licensed relationship therapist, and author of *Doing It: Real People Having Really Good Sex*. Her "Ask Isadora" advice column has appeared in newsweeklies worldwide for more than twenty-five years. Visit her website at www.askisadora.com.

LORI ANAFARTA, MA, LAMFT, is the clinical director and founder of Beyond Diagnosis Counseling, LLC, in St. Paul and Forest Lake, Minnesota. Visit her website at www.Beyond DiagnosisCounseling.com.

MEGAN ANDELLOUX IS a board-certified sexuality educator American Association of Sex Counselors, Educators, and Therapists and sexologist American College of Sexologists who lectures at colleges, works as a gynecological teaching assistant, and runs The Center for Sexual Pleasure and Health in Pawtucket, Rhode Island. Visit her website at www.ohmegan.com.

CHARLES (CHIP) AUGUST is a Personal Growth and Couples Intimacy Coach; host of "Sex, Love & Intimacy," an internet radio show; and author of *Marital Passion: The Sexless Marriage Makeover*. Visit his website at www.chipaugust.com.

ELLEN BARNARD, MSSW, is a sex educator and counselor on topics of aging and sexuality, cancer and sexuality, and facilitating intimacy at the end of life. She is the coowner of A Woman's Touch Sexuality Resource Center, www.sexualityresources.com.

LIBBY BENNETT, PSYD, and GINGER HOLCZER, PSYD, are clinical psychologists and coauthors of *Finding and Revealing Your Sexual Self: A Guide to Communicating about Sex*. Visit their website at www.psychobabbledocs.com.

VIOLET BLUE IS the author and editor of more than a dozen books on sexuality and is a sex educator who lectures at universities and community colleges. Visit her website at www.tinynibbles.com.

SAGE BOLTE, PHD, MSW, LCSW, OSW-C, is an oncology counselor at Life with Cancer, an Inova Health System service in northern Virginia. Visit the website at www.lifewithcancer.org.

STEPHANIE BUEHLER, PSYD, is a licensed psychologist and sex therapist and is director of The Buehler Institute in Irvine, California (www.thebuehlerinstitute.com). Visit her blog about sex and intimacy at www.theblogerotic.com.

MICHAEL CASTLEMAN, MA, is the author of twelve books, including *Great Sex: The Man's Guide to the Secrets of Whole-Body Sensuality* and *Sexual Solutions: For Men and the Women*

Who Love Them. Visit his website about sex after midlife at www
.GreatSexAfter40.com.

MICHELE CAUCH, MA, MSW, is the executive director of Toronto-
based SageHealth Network (www.sagehealthnetwork.com), an
agency promoting seniors' sexual health and positive aging. Visit
her blog at www.seniorsex.blogspot.com.

GLENDA CORWIN, PHD, author of *Sexual Intimacy for Women:
A Guide for Same Sex Couples,* is a clinical psychologist providing gay-affirmative psychotherapy and sexual-intimacy workshops for women who partner with women. Visit her website at
www.drglendacorwin.com.

CAROL DENKER is the author of *Autumn Romance: Stories and
Portraits of Love after 50.* Visit her website at www.autumn
love.org.

BARB DEPREE, MD, is a women's health provider specializing in
menopause care in West Michigan. She founded MiddlesexMD
to help women enjoy sexuality for life, offering clinically sound
information, practical advice, and intimacy aids. Visit her website
at http://MiddlesexMD.com.

JED DIAMOND, PHD, author of *Male Menopause and Mr. Mean:
Saving Your Relationship from the Irritable Male Syndrome,* is a
psychotherapist working with men and women over forty. Visit
his website at www.MenAlive.com.

BETTY DODSON, PHD, artist, author, and sexologist, has been a
voice for women's sexual pleasure and health for more than three
decades. Her books include *Betty Dodson: My Sexual Revolution,*

Sex for One: The Joy of Selfloving, and *Orgasms for Two: The Joy of Partnersex.* Visit her website at www.dodsonandross.com.

DOSSIE EASTON, A longtime player on the San Francisco S/M scene, is coauthor with Janet Hardy of several books on BDSM, including *The Ethical Slut* and *When Someone You Love Is Kinky.* She is a licensed psychotherapist in private practice. Visit her website at www.dossieeaston.com.

YVONNE K. FULBRIGHT, PHD, MSED, is a certified sex educator and the author of several books, including *Sultry Sex Talk to Seduce Any Lover, The Better Sex Guide to Extraordinary Lovemaking,* and *The Hot Guide to Safer Sex.* Visit her websites at www.yvonnekfulbright.com and www.sensualfusion.com.

FRANCESCA GENTILLÉ IS a clinical sexologist, relationship counselor, and contributing author to *The Marriage of Sex & Spirit.* She hosts the Internet radio show "Sex: Tantra & Kama Sutra." Visit her website at www.lifedancecenter.com.

CHARLIE GLICKMAN, PHD, is the Education Program Manager at Good Vibrations (www.goodvibes.com). He offers workshops and classes on a wide range of sexuality topics, including sex-positivity, sex and shame, and sexual diversity and practices.

JOE HANSON IS a life coach, a grief and loss counselor, and the author of *Soaring into Acceptance: Moving through Change and Loss and into Acceptance.* Visit his website at www.lifelessons .info.

GERALD HASLAM IS the author of eighteen books, including *Grace Period*, a novel about prostate cancer, and the editor of eight anthologies. Visit his website at www.geraldhaslam.com.

KEN HASLAM, MD, leads workshops educating senior citizens to be comfortable about their changing sexuality. He is a ten-year polyamory activist who founded a collection of polyamory archives at the Kinsey Institute, Indiana University, Bloomington, Indiana.

DAVID HERSH, MD, is clinical director of The Hersh Centre for Sexual Wellness. He is a sexologist, psychotherapist, and marital therapist in private practice, with offices in Calgary, Alberta; Nelson, British Columbia; and San Francisco, California. Visit his website at www.sexualwellness.ca.

ANNE KATZ, RN, PHD, is the author of *Woman Cancer Sex*, *Man Cancer Sex* and *Breaking the Silence on Cancer and Sexuality: A Handbook for Health Care Providers*. She is the sexuality counselor at CancerCare Manitoba in Canada. Visit her website at www.drannekatz.com.

SUSAN KELLOGG SPADT, PHD, CRNP, is a vulvovaginal pain specialist and Director of Sexual Medicine at the Pelvic and Sexual Health Institute of Philadelphia, www.pelvicandsexualhealth institute.org.

DANIEL KUHN, MSW, is Community Educator for the LIFE Institute of Rainbow Hospice and Palliative Care, www.rainbow hospice.org, based in Park Ridge, Illinois. He has authored or coauthored more than fifty publications, including *Alzheimer's Early Stages: First Steps for Family, Friends and Caregivers*.

ERICA MANFRED, DIVORCED at sixty, is the author of *He's History, You're Not: Surviving Divorce after Forty*. Visit her website at www.heshistory.com.

MICHELE MARSH, PHD, is a certified sex therapist and licensed psychologist practicing at the Council for Relationships (www.councilforrelationships.org) in Wynnewood and Philadelphia, Pennsylvania. She works with people of all ages and uses Eye Movement Desensitization and Reprocessing (EMDR) for trauma resolution.

SUSANA MAYER, PHD, is a board-certified clinical sexologist with a doctorate in human sexuality. Her Ageless Sex Life is a philosophy and program of techniques to assist with sexual drive/desire issues. Visit her website at www.SusanaMayer.com.

LAURIE MINTZ, PHD, is a licensed psychologist, a professor at the University of Missouri, the author of *A Tired Woman's Guide to Passionate Sex: Reclaim Your Desire and Reignite Your Relationship*, and a tired woman who has regained her once-lost passion. Visit her website at www.drlauriemintz.com.

LOREN A. OLSON, MD, is a board-certified clinical psychiatrist recognized as a Distinguished Life Fellow by the American Psychiatric Association. He's also the author of *Finally Out*. Visit his blog for mature gay men at www.magneticfire.com.

LOU PAGET IS the author of five books, including *How to Be a Great Lover* and *How to Give Her Absolute Pleasure*, translated into twenty-eight languages; CEO of Frankly Speaking Inc.; an AASECT-certified sex educator; and a regular media expert on all things sexual. Visit her website at www.loupaget.com.

CAROL QUEEN, PHD, is a writer, speaker, educator, and activist with a doctorate in sexology. She is Staff Sexologist at Good Vibrations (www.goodvibes.com) and founding director of the Center for Sex & Culture (www.sexandculture.org). Visit her website at www.carolqueen.com.

MARNIA ROBINSON IS a science journalist author of *Cupid's Poisoned Arrow: From Habit to Harmony in Sexual Relationships*. Visit her website at www.reuniting.info.

CANDIDA ROYALLE—KNOWN FOR pioneering the genre of woman-friendly erotic films and the Natural Contours line of intimate massagers—is the author of *How to Tell a Naked Man What to Do*. Visit her website at www.candidaroyalle.com.

REBEKAH SKOOR, MA, MS, IMFT, is a professor of Sexuality Studies and Counseling in San Francisco, California. She also counsels individuals, couples, and families, and specializes in relationships and healing from interpersonal trauma. Visit her website at www.rebekahskoor.com.

JEANE TAYLOR, LCSW—A psychotherapist in private practice in Santa Rosa, California—has been helping people for more than thirty years.

TINA B. TESSINA, PHD, also known as Dr. Romance, is a licensed psychotherapist and author of thirteen books, including *How to Be a Couple and Still Be Free* and *The Unofficial Guide to Dating Again*. Visit her website at www.tinatessina.com and her blog at http://drromance.typepad.com/dr_romance_blog.

YOLANDA (LANDI) TURNER, EDD, is a therapist who specializes in online relationships. She is a professor at Eastern University (St. Davids, Pennsylvania) and Widener University (Chester, Pennsylvania). Visit her website at www.drlanditurner.com.

RABBI ED WEINSBERG, EDD, DD, is a prostate-cancer survivor, gerontologist, healthcare and sex educator, and author of *Conquer Prostate Cancer: How Medicine, Faith, Love and Sex Can Renew Your Life,* with Robert Carey, MD. Visit his website at www.ConquerProstateCancer.com.

DIANA WILEY, PHD, is a board-certified sex therapist, clinical sexologist, marriage and family therapist, and gerontologist affiliated with the Seattle Institute for Sex Therapy, Education, and Research. Visit her website at www.DrDianaWiley.com.

MYRTLE WILHITE, MD, MS, is a physician and epidemiologist who specializes in prevention strategies to help maintain sexual health and wellness. She is the coowner of A Woman's Touch Sexuality Resource Center (www.sexualityresources.com).

ACKNOWLEDGMENTS

I AM GRATEFUL TO all of you who contributed your stories to *Naked at Our Age* by sending me your interviews, concerns, and questions. Without your candor and willingness to share your intimate experiences, this book could not have been written.

I am indebted to the experts who generously addressed my readers' concerns (and mine!) and contributed their sage advice for making senior sex better.

I thank the wonderful folks at Seal Press who believed wholeheartedly in the mission of this book and made the whole process a delight for me (as they did with *Better Than I Ever Expected: Straight Talk about Sex after Sixty*)—especially my editor, Brooke Warner, and Seal's publicist, Andie East.

I thank in advance those people who will ridicule our desire for lifelong sexuality, because they will spur us to speak out even more loudly!

ABOUT THE AUTHOR

A UTHOR AND SPEAKER Joan Price calls herself an "advocate for ageless sexuality." At age sixty-one, Joan wrote *Better Than I Ever Expected: Straight Talk about Sex after Sixty* (Seal Press, 2006) to celebrate the delights of older-life sexuality—especially her spicy love affair with artist Robert Rice, who became her husband. She followed that book up five years later with *Naked at Our Age: Talking Out Loud about Senior Sex* after hundreds of readers sent her questions about improving their own senior sex lives.

Formerly a high school English teacher, Joan is also a fitness professional and author of *The Anytime, Anywhere Exercise Book: 300+ Quick and Easy Exercises You Can Do Whenever You Want*. Joan teaches contemporary line dancing (which she calls "the most fun you can have with both feet on the floor") in Sebastopol and Santa Rosa, California.

Visit Joan's website at www.joanprice.com and her zesty blog about sex and aging at www.NakedAtOurAge.com.

NOTES

CHAPTER 1

1   Stacy Tessler Lindau and Natalia Gavrilova, "Sex, Health, and Years of Sexually Active Life Gained due to Good Health: Evidence from Two US Population Based Cross Sectional Surveys of Ageing," *British Medical Journal*, 340 (2010): c810.

CHAPTER 11

1   The Vaginal Renewal program can be found at the website http://bit.ly/vrprogarticle.

CHAPTER 12

1   More information from the National Cancer Institute can be found at the website www.cancer.gov/cancertopics /life-after-treatment/page5#d2.

CHAPTER 19

1   Linda L. Fisher et al., "Sex, Romance, and Relationships: AARP Survey of Midlife and Older Adults" (Washington, DC: AARP), http://assets.aarp.org/rgcenter/general/srr_09 .pdf, p. 30.

2   Centers for Disease Control and Prevention website, www .cdc.gov/hiv/topics/over50 (accessed September 5, 2010).

3   National Institute on Aging website, www.nia.nih.gov/ HealthInformation/Publications/hiv-aids.htm (accessed September 5, 2010).

4   Stacy Tessler Lindau et al., "Older Women's Attitudes, Behavior, and Communication about Sex and HIV: A Community-Based Study," *Journal of Women's Health* 15, no. 6 (2006). Available at www.cbs.com/cbs_cares/topics/ HIV_Older_Women.pdf (accessed September 5, 2010).

5   The Body website, www.thebody.com/content/art6036.html (accessed September 5, 2010).

6   Travis I. Lovejoy et al., "Patterns and Correlates of Sexual Activity and Condom Use Behavior in Persons 50-Plus Years of Age Living with HIV/AIDS," *AIDS and Behavior* 12, no. 6 (2008): 943–956.

7   Centers for Disease Control and Prevention website, www.cdc.gov/hiv/topics/over50/challenges.htm (accessed September 5, 2010).

INDEX

as hormonal, 38; manual. *See*
manual arousal; pelvic floor
as relaxed by, 181–182; post-
cancer, 202; psychological,
35; self-pleasuring as serving,
145–146; slowing, 28, 40–41,
220; vigorous penile stimulation,
236; whole-bodily, 254; without
reproductive hormones, 27;
youthful signs of, 24
arthritis, 15
assumptions, 81, 83
attraction: feeling sexy, 42–44;
of young men to older women,
114–115
August, Chip, 24
*Autumn Romance: Stories and
Portraits of Love after 50*
(Denker), 321
AwakeningBody.com, 301

B
bacterial vaginosis, 174
ball rings, 56
barbell, vaginal, 141–142
Barnard MSSW, Ellen: on abuse,
74; on change in arousal, 40;
reasons to maintain sex life,
139–140; on sharing sexual
needs, 84; on vaginal pain, 173,
176; vaginal therapy tips, 181,
183; on women's orgasmic
difficulty, 32; on women's
pleasure, 17
BDSM (Bondage and Discipline,
Sadism and Masochism), 107–
114
Bennet, PSYD, Libby, 87–88, 246
betrayal, 131–136
*Better Than I Ever Expected:
Straight Talk about Sex After
Sixty* (Price): for doctors, 192;
erection education in, 281;
overcoming embarassment

to write, 52; Robert Rice as
inspiring, 5, 305; senior sex as
celebrated in, 345; testimonials
to, 237, 284; Vaginal Renewal
program, 189
blood flow, 28, 30, 40, 341
blood tests, for STDs, 333
Blue, Violet, 61–62
body language, 83
Bolte, Sage, 200–203
bonding: with daily snuggles,
358–359; in long-term
relationships, 353–359; sensory,
286; sexual, 197–198
booty calls, 106–107
boundaries, 109–111, 113
break ups: after an affair,
135–136; allowing for grief,
123–126; counseling for, 32;
initiating, 75–78
breast cancer, 208–209
breast touch, 9–10
breath, 39
British Medical Journal, 16, 17
Britton, Dr. Patti, 233–234
Buehler, PSYD, Stephanie, 214
butt plugs, 56

C
cancer, 197–218; breast,
208–209; life-affirmation after,
197–198; reclaiming sex after,
214; of Robert Rice, 172, 197;
sex as healing tool, 210–214;
tips for sex after, 200–203; *see
also* prostate cancer
caregiving, 262, 287
caressing, 37, 39, 103, 208,
225–226
Castleman, MA., Michael, 13, 96,
223, 235, 244, 248
casual sex, 106–107
Cauch, Michele, 314, 336–337
celibacy: following spouse's death,

188; and "revirgination", 180,
181; solo sex during, 141–142
Centers for Disease Control and
Prevention (CDC), 327, 330
change, in arousals: allowing,
24; communicating, 9–10;
with ED, 228; focus away
from intercourse, 163; joy of
older-age sex, 347–353; for
men, 147; noticing, 40–41;
post-reproducive-hormone,
27; reasons for, 12; sudden, as
medical concern, 28; ups and
downs with, 8
choice, 95
clitoris: education on, 149;
lubrication of, 21; stimulation
to orgasm, 145–146, 231–234,
235; vibrator stimulation of,
50–51
cock rings, 56, 58–59, 341
communication, 79–96; about
cancer, 213–216, 249; about
changing responses, 9–10; about
erectile dysfunction, 244–248;
about low desire, 46; about need
for counseling, 91; about sexual
limits, 240; about sexual needs,
66, 72, 80; about vaginal pain,
176–177, 179; choosing times
for, 87; examples, 10–11; gentle,
80; healthy, principles of, 81;
honest, 10, 39–40; importance
of, 41; in polyamorous
relationships, 98, 101; post-
cancer, 202; post prostate
surgery, 200; secrets and shame,
84–85; sex as aided by good,
89–90; tips, 66, 82–83, 87–88,
246–247
compliments, 171, 270, 319, 359
compulsive behavior, 78
condoms: discussing, 334–335,
337; eroticizing, 147, 339;

female, 338; insisting on, 341–
343; to prevent pregnancy, 169;
to prevent STDs, 326; tips for
use, 336–337, 340–341
consensual BDSM, 111
control, loss of, 265–267
Corwin, PhD., Glenda, 130, 314,
354–355
counseling. See therapy
Craigslist, 295
cuddling, 208, 215, 226, 358–359
cunnilingus. See oral sex
cybersex, 121
cystitis, 174

D

dance class, 277–278, 284
dangers, of paid sex, 295
date rape, 156
dates, sex, 23, 85
dating, 305–323; after breakups,
128–130; communicating
sexual limitations in, 240; after
death of a spouse, 278–279;
handling rejection, 318; how to
meet people, 305; online, 129,
307–313, 314; saying "no",
319–321; as a senior, 104;
success stories, 321–323; women
discuss online, 310–313; worst
first dates, 313–314
Davis, Bette, 3
death of a spouse: in the author's
case, 198; celibacy following,
188; grief counseling, 273–276;
relationships after, 278–279;
sudden, 282
dementia, 259–271
Denker, Carol, 321–322
Depree, MD., Barb, 47–48
depression, 124, 140, 277
desire: and action, 35, 36;
differing, 63–75; faking, 39–41;
increasing, 27–48; and loss of

exercise: as aid to grief, 125, 130; pelvic floor. *See* pelvic floor muscles

experience: benefits of older-age sex, 347–353; in relationship, 116

F

faking it, 39–41, 45

fantasies: in abusive relationship, 73; acting on, 353; BDSM, 108, 109; communicating, 99; erection via, 224; to increase libido, 37–38; permission to own, 155; women as nurturing, 18

farting, 210

fault-finding, 82

FC2 female condom, 338

fear: of pregnancy, 152; of rape, 159

Femme Productions, 140

fingers, arousal with. *See* manual arousal

fitness, pelvic floor, 85

Fleiss, Heidi, 294

food, sex and, 62

foreplay: 24-hour, 354–355; to aid vaginal pain, 180; during condom donning, 339; for consensual BDSM, 111; as education, 171; essentials of, 38–39; lubrication as, 20; phone sex as lacking, 120; sensate focus excercises, 37; on sex dates, 23; taking time for, 145; toys for, 54

friends: with benefits, 106–107, 335; support from, 125

Fulbright, PhD, MSED., Yvonne K., 82

furniture, sex, 16

G

gangbanging, 104–105

gay relationships: for aging men, 310; dating warning signs, 316–317; lesbian dating, 314–315; online dating, 310; waning sexual interest in, 31

gay sex: erectile concerns, 241–242; homophobia about, 154; post-cancer, 217

gender identity change, 12

generational inhibitions, 25

Gentillé, Francesca, 38–39, 71

Getting Naked Again (Sills), 284

Glickman, PhD., Charlie, 58–59, 340

GoodCleanLove.com, 186

Grace Period, 205

grief: of breakups, 123–124; counseling for, 273–276; erectile dysfuction from, 229; honoring process of, 124–125, 130; stories of healing from, 279–289

Growing Up, 156

G-spot, 211

guidance, lack of, 159–160

guilt, 103, 151, 166

gynecological exams, 181, 192

H

Halperin, Sherry, 313

Hanson, Joe, 274–276

The Happy Hooker (Hollander), 152

Haslam, Gerald, 206

Haslam, MD, Ken, 93, 100–101

health: arousal as aided by, 28; of pelvic floor muscles, 70; of self-pleasure, 74, 137–138; sex life as aiding, 47–48, 102; STD risk for seniors, 326–327; tools for, 17; vaginal, 139, 141, 201

heart disease, 29

Hersh, MD., David, 222, 358

muscles, 182; tips for, 231–234; and vaginal health, 139

marriage: education, 95; for immigration reasons, 118–119; lack of education in, 154–155; open, 97–104; rebound, 151; sexless, 63–75; *see also* relationships

Marsh, PhD., Michele, 68

massage: hired erotic, 291–293, 300–303; sensual, for men, 253–254; vaginal, 183–184, 187, 190–191

masturbation, 137–148; for boys, 162; cock rings for, 59; with condoms, 340; education, 166; exploring, 71; as foundational, 1–2; during grieving, 278; health of, 139–142; for men, 146–148, 166; partner-assisted, 3; partner's reaction to, 73; post-cancer, 203; reasons for, 138–139; as "research", 41, 42, 88, 145–146; shared, 143–144, 211, 237–238; talking about, 52; toys for, 52–53; via webcam, 115, 117, 119–121; women's workshops on, 143

Mead, Margaret, 2

Meet Our Experts section, 8

men: information on sex for, 5; masturbation for, 144, 146–148; overcoming manhood norms, 161–172; response to ED, 244–245; sensual massage for, 253–254

menopause: "male", 162; as a new beginning, 2; and pelvic floor tension, 181–182; pelvic floor weakening after, 141

mindfulness, 36–37

Mintz, PhD., Laurie, 45–46, 65, 81

missionary position, 143–144, 207

money, love and, 126–128

monogamy, 98, 107

multipartner sex, 104–106

myeloma, 212

N

NakedAtOurAge.com, 8, 53, 196, 306

Naked at Our Age: Talking Out Loud about Senior Sex (Price), 7

nakedness, 67, 103, 217

National Cancer Institute, 215–216

Natural Contours Énergie vaginal barbell, 141

Naughty Boy, 59

nonoxynol-9, 61

non-traditional sex practices, 97–121

O

oil-based lubricants, 21

Olson, MD., Loren A., 220

online sex, 115, 117, 119–121

oral sex: expressing desire for, 92–93; for men without erections, 208, 257; pornography combined with, 11; positions to aid, 15; tips for, 231–234; women's preference for, 225

orgasm: avoiding big, 147; cock ring effects on, 58; creating vs. allowing, 13–14; from cunnilingus, 231–234; drab, 13, 14; enjoyment of partners', 11; healthiness of, 50, 139–140, 184, 191; as "in the moment", 37; longer time to achieve, 145, 147; maintaining regular, 18, 28, 32–33; masturbation for, 143–144; medications preventing, 32, 57; self-pleasuring "research" on,

Viagra, 237–239, 246, 263–264
vibrators: as added arousal
   source, 14; guilt about, 50;
   lubricating, 57–58; myths and
   facts about, 50–52; orgasm via,
   146; for partner sex, 54–55; for
   solo sex, 52–53; vaginal massage
   with, 191
virginity, losing, 167
vulvodynia, 174

W
water-based lubricants, 21
weight gain, 85
Weinsberg, Rabbi Ed, 226
widowhood: vs. breakup, 123;
   solo sex in, 52; *see also* death of
   a spouse; grief
Wiley, PhD., Diana, 36–38
Wilhite, MD., Myrtle, 30, 187,
   190–191

wisdom, 347–353
women: early life pleasure
   education, 138; on ED, 243–
   257; as at fault for rape, 158;
   lack of desire in, 43, 46; orgasm
   from intercourse, 235; sex as
   done "to", 92; sexual pleasure
   aids, 17; unlearning sexual mis-
   education, 149–160
World of Warcraft, 115

Y
yeast infections, 62, 194
Your Perfect Right (Alberti and
   Emmons), 69

Z
Zoloft, 124

SELECTED TITLES FROM SEAL PRESS

For more than thirty years, Seal Press has published groundbreaking books. By women. For women.

Better Than I Ever Expected: Straight Talk about Sex after Sixty, by Joan Price. $15.95, 978-1-58005-152-1. A warm, witty, and honest book that contends with the challenges and celebrates the delights of older-life sexuality.

Free Fall: A Late-in-Life Love Affair, by Rae Padilla Francoeur. $16.95, 978-1-58005-304-4. In this erotic memoir, Rae Padilla Francoeur recounts the joys, benefits, and challenges of embarking upon a surprising love affair late in life, and inspires women over fifty to discover their deepest sexual self.

For Keeps: Women Tell the Truth about Their Bodies, Growing Older, and Acceptance, edited by Victoria Zackheim. $15.95, 978-1-58005-204-7. This inspirational collection of personal essays explores the relationship that aging women have with their bodies.

Rescue Me, He's Wearing a Moose Hat: And 40 Other Dates after 50, by Sherry Halperin. $13.95, 978-1-58005-068-5. The hilarious account of a woman who finds herself back in the dating scene after midlife.

Sexual Intimacy for Women: A Guide for Same-Sex Couples, by Glenda Corwin, Ph.D. $16.95, 978-1-58005-303-7. In this prescriptive and poignant book, Glenda Corwin, PhD, helps female couples overcome obstacles to sexual intimacy through her examination of the emotional, physical, and psychological aspects of same-sex relationships.

Dear John, I Love Jane: Women Write about Leaving Men for Women, edited by Candance Walsh and Laura André. $16.95, 978-1-58005-339-6. A timely collection of stories that are sometimes funny and sometimes painful—but always achingly honest—accounts of leaving a man for a woman, and the consequences of making such a choice.

FIND SEAL PRESS ONLINE
www.SealPress.com
www.Facebook.com/SealPress
Twitter: @SealPress